# Your Guide to
# Alternative
# MEDICINE

## Understanding, Locating, and Selecting
## Holistic Treatments and Practitioners

# Larry P. Credit
# Sharon G. Hartunian
# Margaret J. Nowak

**SQUAREONE**
P U B L I S H E R S

COVER DESIGNER: Phaedra Mastrocola
IN-HOUSE EDITOR: Elaine Kennedy and Helene Ciaravino
TYPESETTER: Gary A. Rosenberg
COVER PHOTOS: Getty Images, Inc.


**Square One Publishers**
115 Herricks Road
Garden City Park, NY 11040
(516) 535-2010 • (877) 900-BOOK
www.squareonepublishers.com



**Library of Congress Cataloging-in-Publication Data**

Credit, Larry P.
  Your guide to alternative medicine : understanding, locating, and
selecting holistic treatments and practitioners / Larry P. Credit,
Sharon G. Hartunian, Margaret J. Nowak.
    p. cm.
  Includes bibliographical references and index.
  ISBN 0-7570-0125-4 (pbk.)
  1. Alternative medicine—Popular works.  I. Hartunian, Sharon G.
II. Nowak, Margaret J.  III. Title.
R733 .C7348 2003
615.5—dc22

                                              2003015376

Printed in the United States of America

10   9   8   7   6   5   4   3   2   1

# Contents

*We dedicate this book to our parents and our children,
for their unceasing support, understanding, and patience
during the writing process.*

*To our parents, who are of the generation that survived
the first Genocide of this century, the Great Depression,
and the World Wars, we thank you for opening your hearts
and minds to our voices, even when our life choices
and work interests were not the norm.*

*To our children, Talyn, Sara, and Cali,
we thank you for your endless energy, boundless joy,
and constant needs that kept us connected to life's true priorities.
You have enriched our lives with love.*

*With this book, we hope to enrich the lives of others
with an awareness of the opportunities for healthy living.*

# Acknowledgments

We would like to acknowledge the astute and ongoing support, suggestions, and guidance given to us by Rudy Shur and Helene Ciaravino of Square One Publishers. Their navigational leadership, from rough manuscript to polished book, was greatly appreciated and unquestionably valuable. We would also like to acknowledge our colleagues in alternative medicine who have shared their expertise and skills with us throughout our careers. Thank you for opening up windows of possibilities in the realm of healthcare.

# Introduction

James Reston, correspondent to *The New York Times*, was visiting China in the hot summer of 1971. An attack of acute appendicitis forced him into the Anti-Imperialist Hospital in Peking. Reston detailed the significant experience that followed in a groundbreaking front-page article which appeared in *The New York Times*. He described an "intensely human and vibrant" atmosphere in which his medical emergency was deftly treated with a mixture of conventional medical practices and ancient Chinese healing arts. A local anesthetic was used to numb Reston's mid-section, and surgery was performed. He remained conscious throughout the procedure, which was completed with "no complications, nausea or vomiting." For post-surgical pain and discomfort, Reston received acupuncture and herbal medicine. These alternative medicine treatments resulted in "a noticeable relaxation of the pressure and distension [of the stomach] . . . and no recurrence of the problem thereafter." With the appearance of this story, our nation was awakened to alternative medicine through a media voice that announced the healing potential of medical treatments that combine the "very old with the very new."

In the same spirit of optimism and respect for the pairing of conventional and holistic/wholistic medicine, we have endeavored to introduce you to a number of alternative medicine approaches, so that you, too, can benefit from healthcare that encompasses current science and technology *and* the wisdom of the ages. We recognize that in order to encourage consumers of healthcare to try alternative medicine approaches, we must describe the treatments in a clear, direct manner, and then lay out the practical steps toward finding a trained practitioner.

This handbook is the key to understanding alternative medicine options. Our goal is to give you the basic facts and practical guidance necessary to choose an appropriate therapy and to successfully initiate treatment. In an easy-to-read, quick-referencing format, this text covers the following topics for each alternative medicine approach:

- *What Is It?:* a brief description and history of the approach.

- *Conditions That Respond Best:* what conditions are usually treated by this approach.

- *How Does It Work?:* the philosophy and procedures followed during therapy.

- *What to Expect:* what you will encounter when being treated.

- *Cost/Duration:* average cost and time ranges for treatment sessions.

- *Credentials/Education:* what you should consider regarding the background and training of practitioners.

- *How to Find a Practitioner:* the best ways to contact a practitioner.

- *Professional Organizations:* groups that are involved in disseminating information about the approach, licensing or certifying practitioners, and providing training and/or referrals.

- *Recommended Reading:* suggested resources for further information and study.

Alternative medicine, commonly referred to as *holistic* or *wholistic* healthcare, covers treatment options that generally are not a part of conventional medical practice. These approaches are viewed as *complements to conventional Western medicine.* In partnership with conventional medicine, the treatments can bolster your potential for health and recovery. It is clear that when it comes to emergency procedures and appropriate surgical interventions, conventional medicine excels. However, a combination of standard treatments and alternative medicine approaches can be very effective.

The belief that the mind influences the body and that the body, in turn, has an impact on the mind is a key element in the philosophy of alternative medicine. As a result, alternative medicine focuses on the health needs of the whole person. Practitioners strive to be aware of their clients' health from a number of perspectives; physical, emotional, nutritional, and spiritual factors are considered. The emphasis of treatment is on the body's ability to heal itself with the help of natural, non-invasive therapies that are effective and without harmful side effects.

Alternative medicine supports client education and encourages positive lifestyle changes. Practitioners serve dual roles as treatment specialists and teachers. They work in partnership with their clients, motivating them toward better health and helping to strengthen the internal healing potential of each individual.

Sometimes, terms used to describe alternative medicine can be confusing because of their holistic context. For example, *balance,* in holistic terms, refers to the equality between the body and the mind—both have equal influence on your health and both must operate optimally in order to minimize dysfunction. Likewise, the term *harmony* refers to the facile interaction of the systems of the body and mind. Restoring balance and harmony are often goals of alternative medicine. To assist you in better understanding alternative medicine approaches, we have provided the definitions of essential terms in the glossary.

While alternative medicine approaches are helpful for individuals experiencing chronic pain and seriously debilitating disorders, they also benefit those who are interested in maintaining health and preventing future problems. You do not need an illness or an injury to be treated. Just as a well-oiled machine functions smoothly, the magnificent human body operates at its best when cared for on a regular basis with health-enhancing regimens.

The overall goal of alternative medicine is to put your well-being into your own hands, so that you become an active participant in your recovery and/or health maintenance. We have researched approaches thoroughly and have interviewed numerous practitioners in our quest to bring you a concise, accessible handbook. Our hope is that you will consider this book a trusted guide to the healing realm of alternative medicine.

Please note that throughout this book, we refer to practitioners according to their education, certificates, and degrees. For example, a chiropractor is also a *doctor,* and is therefore termed as such in various places. As we work to popularize alternative care approaches, we also endeavor to erase the various stereotypes and prejudices that have formed around them. Practitioners of alternative medicine accomplish much study in, and exhibit tremendous commitment to, their chosen practices. We hope that the public will become increasingly comfortable using titles that properly refer to professionals who have trained so diligently in their specialties.

## GUIDELINES FOR CHOOSING A THERAPY

In order to be a successful navigator of your own healthcare, it is important to know your treatment goals and personal inclinations, as well as the professional background, experience, and manner of the practitioner. The following guidelines offer helpful advice on how to go about deciding on an alternative medicine program.

### Considering Various Treatments

When researching alternative medicine options, keep in mind the following pointers:

- *Remain open.* Welcome the opportunity to try something different. Accept the norm as but one solution to the puzzle, and expand your options to the unfamiliar.

- *Determine your goals.* What do you want to receive from alternative medicine? Whether you consider yourself healthy and wish to maintain this health, or you have an acute condition that you would rather live without, setting goals will act as a guide in choosing an approach.

- *Explore.* Investigate the various approaches and find the ones that best suit your goals. Build confidence by making new choices through knowledge. The more you know, the more control you have.

- *Determine your comfort level.* After exploring your options and finding appropriate treatments, shorten the list by assessing how comfortable you are with each approach. For example, while acupuncture, massage, and Therapeutic Touch are all treatments that can focus on eliminating headaches, each has its own method. Select the approach that is the best match for *you.* Remember to remain open. Often, comfort level increases as treatments progress and trust is established.

## Choosing a Practitioner

When selecting a treatment specialist, consider the following suggestions so that you will find a practitioner who matches your expectations and needs:

- *Take your time.* Gather the names of practitioners by using the various sources available to you: for a referral in your area, contact the professional organizations listed at the end of each approach section in this book; get a recommendation from someone whose opinion you respect; look in your local yellow pages under the suggested categories in our *How to Find a Practitioner* sections. Call the practitioners and ask questions about their schooling, how long they have been practicing, and what their current licensing or certification is. Inquire about their fees, their general procedures with a new client, and their experience in treating your specific condition. Do not let yourself be pressured into setting up an appointment; have them send you a brochure. Explain that you are in the process of gathering information and are not ready to make a commitment.

- *Review the information.* Because you have done your research, you will be able to quickly assess if the practitioner has the proper qualifications. When making a final decision, carefully review all of the information that you have gathered, and keep the total package in mind. How were the practitioners' phone manners? Did they sound professional? Were they willing to talk about their educational backgrounds and treatment procedures? Are you comfortable with their qualifications? Did they have standard fees or were they hesitant to discuss money?

Because it is important to feel at ease with a practitioner, it may be wise to have an initial consultation with him or her before making a final decision. Trust your judgment concerning your confidence in the skills and personal manner of each practitioner so that, upon final selection, an optimal healing relationship can be established.

- *Use the first appointment as an evaluation.* Approach the appointment with your goals clearly established. Review these goals with the practitioner and organize a treatment plan. The program should be well-focused, allowing you to budget your time and expenses while guiding you in attaining your goals. Discuss possible side effects and/or adverse reactions. Do not be afraid to ask questions. Remember that you are in charge.

## Evaluating Your Experience

After a consultation and/or treatment session, fill out the following assessment form. The results will provide a concise, focused critique of the treatment specialist.

| *During my treatment session, I felt that I was provided with:* | ABOVE AVERAGE | AVERAGE | BELOW AVERAGE |
|---|---|---|---|
| • Adequate information regarding diagnosis, tests, treatment, progress, and prognosis. | ❏ | ❏ | ❏ |
| • The opportunity to participate in setting treatment goals. | ❏ | ❏ | ❏ |
| • Treatment that was designed according to my needs. | ❏ | ❏ | ❏ |
| • An appropriate home program (if applicable). | ❏ | ❏ | ❏ |

| *Did my therapist make the grade for:* | | | |
|---|---|---|---|
| • Promptness | ❏ | ❏ | ❏ |
| • Professionalism | ❏ | ❏ | ❏ |
| • Willingness to answer questions | ❏ | ❏ | ❏ |
| • Willingness to listen | ❏ | ❏ | ❏ |
| • Understanding my concerns | ❏ | ❏ | ❏ |

# Quick-Reference Table

The following quick-reference table suggests a number of alternative medicine approaches to consider when seeking treatment for a particular type of condition. Each listed approach is discussed at length in its own section of this book.

| TYPE OF CONDITION | APPROPRIATE ALTERNATIVE MEDICINE APPROACHES |
|---|---|
| **Allergy** | Acupressure; Acupuncture; Ayurveda; Chiropractic; Flower Essences; Foot Reflexology; Herbal Medicine; Holistic Dentistry; Homeopathy; Lymphatic Massage; Naturopathy; Nutritional Counseling; Polarity Therapy; Shiatsu; Traditional Chinese Medicine |
| **Back Pain** | Acupressure; Acupuncture; Alexander Technique; Aquatic Therapy; Aromatherapy; Ayurveda; Biofeedback; Chiropractic; CranioSacral Therapy; Feldenkrais Method; Foot Reflexology; Hatha Yoga; Herbal Medicine; Homeopathy; Hypnotherapy; Naturopathy; Nutritional Counseling; Polarity Therapy; Psychotherapy; Qigong; Reiki; Relaxation/Meditation; Rolfing; Shiatsu; Sports Massage; Swedish Massage; Tai Chi; Therapeutic Touch; Traditional Chinese Medicine; Trager Approach; Trigger Point Therapy |
| **Balance/ Coordination Disorder** | Acupressure; Acupuncture; Alexander Technique; Aquatic Therapy; Aromatherapy; Ayurveda; Chiropractic; Cranio-Sacral Therapy; Feldenkrais Method; Foot Reflexology; Hatha Yoga; Herbal Medicine; Homeopathy; Naturopathy; Nutritional Counseling; Polarity Therapy; Qigong; Reiki; |

| | |
|---|---|
| | Relaxation/Meditation; Rolfing; Shiatsu; Tai Chi; Traditional Chinese Medicine; Trager Approach |
| **Cardio-vascular Disorder** | Acupressure; Acupuncture; Aquatic Therapy; Ayurveda; Biofeedback; Foot Reflexology; Hatha Yoga; Herbal Medicine; Homeopathy; Hypnotherapy; Naturopathy; Nutritional Counseling; Polarity Therapy; Psychotherapy; Qigong; Relaxation/Meditation; Shiatsu; Swedish Massage; Tai Chi; Traditional Chinese Medicine; Trager Approach |
| **Circulatory Disorder** | Acupressure; Acupuncture; Alexander Technique; Aquatic Therapy; Aromatherapy; Ayurveda; Biofeedback; Foot Reflexology; Hatha Yoga; Herbal Medicine; Homeopathy; Hypnotherapy; Naturopathy; Nutritional Counseling; Polarity Therapy; Qigong; Relaxation/Meditation; Rolfing; Shiatsu; Sports Massage; Swedish Massage; Tai Chi; Traditional Chinese Medicine; Trager Approach; Trigger Point Therapy |
| **Dermatological Condition** | Acupressure; Acupuncture; Aromatherapy; Ayurveda; Flower Essences; Foot Reflexology; Herbal Medicine; Homeopathy; Naturopathy; Nutritional Counseling; Polarity Therapy; Relaxation/Meditation; Shiatsu; Traditional Chinese Medicine |
| **Digestive Disorder** | Acupressure; Acupuncture; Aromatherapy; Ayurveda; Biofeedback; Chiropractic; Flower Essences; Foot Reflexology; Hatha Yoga; Nutritional Counseling; Polarity Therapy; Qigong; Relaxation/Meditation; Rolfing; Shiatsu; Swedish Massage; Tai Chi; Traditional Chinese Medicine; Trager Approach |
| **Eating Disorder** | Acupressure; Acupuncture; Aromatherapy; Ayurveda; Biofeedback; Flower Essences; Herbal Medicine; Hypnotherapy; Naturopathy; Nutritional Counseling; Polarity Therapy; Psychotherapy; Relaxation/Meditation; Traditional Chinese Medicine |
| **Emotional Health Disorder (including stress/anxiety)** | Acupressure; Acupuncture; Alexander Technique, Aquatic Therapy; Aromatherapy; Ayurveda; Biofeedback; Cranio-Sacral Therapy; Feldenkrais Method; Flower Essences; Foot Reflexology; Hatha Yoga; Herbal Medicine; Holistic Dentistry; Homeopathy; Hypnotherapy; Naturopathy; Nutritional |

| | |
|---|---|
| | Counseling; Polarity Therapy; Psychotherapy; Qigong; Reiki; Relaxation/Meditation; Rolfing; Shiatsu; Swedish Massage; Tai Chi; Therapeutic Touch; Traditional Chinese Medicine; Trager Approach; Trigger Point Therapy |
| **Endocrine Disorder** | Acupressure; Acupuncture; Aromatherapy; Ayurveda; Chiropractic; Flower Essences; Foot Reflexology; Herbal Medicine; Homeopathy; Hypnotherapy; Naturopathy; Nutritional Counseling; Polarity Therapy; Shiatsu; Traditional Chinese Medicine; Trager Approach |
| **Eye, Ear, Nose, Throat Condition** | Acupressure; Acupuncture; Alexander Technique; Aromatherapy; Ayurveda; Chiropractic; CranioSacral Therapy; Foot Reflexology; Herbal Medicine; Holistic Dentistry; Homeopathy; Naturopathy; Nutritional Counseling; Shiatsu; Traditional Chinese Medicine |
| **Immune Disorder** | Acupressure; Acupuncture; Ayurveda; Biofeedback; Flower Essences; Foot Reflexology; Hatha Yoga; Herbal Medicine; Homeopathy; Lymphatic Massage; Naturopathy; Nutritional Counseling; Polarity Therapy; Psychotherapy; Qigong; Reiki; Relaxation/Meditation; Shiatsu; Swedish Massage; Tai Chi; Therapeutic Touch; Traditional Chinese Medicine; Trager Approach |
| **Musculoskeletal Disorder** | Acupressure; Acupuncture; Alexander Technique; Aquatic Therapy; Aromatherapy; Ayurveda; Biofeedback; Chiropractic; CranioSacral Therapy; Feldenkrais Method; Foot Reflexology; Hatha Yoga; Herbal Medicine; Homeopathy; Hypnotherapy; Naturopathy; Nutritional Counseling; Polarity Therapy; Psychotherapy; Qigong; Reiki; Relaxation/Meditation; Rolfing; Shiatsu; Sports Massage; Swedish Massage; Tai Chi; Therapeutic Touch; Traditional Chinese Medicine; Trager Approach; Trigger Point Therapy |
| **Nervous System Disorder** | Acupressure; Acupuncture; Alexander Technique; Aromatherapy; Ayurveda; Biofeedback; Chiropractic; CranioSacral Therapy; Feldenkrais Method; Flower Essences; Foot Reflexology; Hatha Yoga; Herbal Medicine; Holistic Dentistry; Homeopathy; Hypnotherapy; |

| | |
|---|---|
| | Naturopathy; Nutritional Counseling; Polarity Therapy; Psychotherapy; Qigong; Reiki; Relaxation/Meditation; Rolfing; Shiatsu; Swedish Massage; Tai Chi; Therapeutic Touch; Traditional Chinese Medicine; Trager Approach |
| **Reproductive Disorder** | Acupressure; Acupuncture; Aromatherapy; Ayurveda; Foot Reflexology; Herbal Medicine; Homeopathy; Hypnotherapy; Naturopathy; Nutritional Counseling; Polarity Therapy; Qigong; Reiki; Relaxation/Meditation; Swedish Massage; Traditional Chinese Medicine |
| **Respiratory Disorder** | Acupressure; Acupuncture; Alexander Technique; Aquatic Therapy; Aromatherapy; Ayurveda; Biofeedback; Chiropractic; Feldenkrais Method; Flower Essences; Foot Reflexology; Hatha Yoga; Herbal Medicine; Homeopathy; Hypnotherapy; Naturopathy; Nutritional Counseling; Polarity Therapy; Qigong; Reiki; Relaxation/Meditation; Rolfing; Shiatsu; Swedish Massage; Tai Chi; Traditional Chinese Medicine; Trager Approach |
| **Substance Abuse** | Acupuncture; Ayurveda; Biofeedback; Flower Essences; Herbal Medicine; Homeopathy; Hypnotherapy; Naturopathy; Nutritional Counseling; Psychotherapy; Reiki; Relaxation/Meditation; Therapeutic Touch; Traditional Chinese Medicine |
| **Teeth/Jaw Condition** | Acupressure; Acupuncture; Alexander Technique; Ayurveda; Biofeedback; CranioSacral Therapy; Herbal Medicine; Holistic Dentistry; Homeopathy; Hypnotherapy; Naturopathy; Nutritional Counseling; Relaxation/Meditation; Traditional Chinese Medicine; Trigger Point Therapy |

# A-to-Z Guide to Alternative Medicine

## ACUPRESSURE

### WHAT IS IT?

Acupressure is the application of pressure, using fingers, thumbs, palms, or elbows, to stimulate, disperse, and regulate the body's healing energy. It is an approach based on the philosophies of Traditional Chinese Medicine (see page 151). Over many centuries, through trial and error, the Chinese developed a treatment system that uses the body's natural abilities. The main concept behind this system is that healing energy—*chi*—circulates throughout the body along specific pathways, called *meridians.* The flow of chi through the meridians connects all areas of the body much like the streets on a road map link various locations. It is possible, for example, to treat facial pain by applying pressure to a specific section of the hand, because a meridian connects the two areas.

The goal of Traditional Chinese Medicine is to keep the body in balance and harmony through the free flow of chi. Disease is a result of blockages in this energy current. Acupressure releases chi obstructions through the application of pressure at certain points along the meridians.

### CONDITIONS THAT RESPOND BEST

Acupressure is an appropriate treatment option for the relief or reduction of the following conditions:

- Allergies
- Anxiety
- Arthritis
- Asthma
- Back pain
- Bronchitis

- Carpal tunnel syndrome, wrist pain
- Chronic fatigue
- Colic
- Constipation
- Depression
- Disc problems
- Dizziness
- Eating disorders
- Fibroids
- Foot, ankle pain
- Hay fever
- Headaches, migraines
- Hormonal imbalance
- Hyper-, hypotension
- Immune system weakness
- Indigestion
- Knee, hip, pelvic pain
- Neck, shoulder pain
- Neuralgia
- Poor circulation
- Premenstrual syndrome (pms)
- Restricted breathing
- Rheumatism
- Sciatica
- Sinus problems
- Skin problems
- Sleep disorders
- Stress
- Swollen lymph nodes
- Temporomandibular joint (TMJ) syndrome
- Tennis elbow
- Ulcers
- Varicose veins
- Water retention

## HOW DOES IT WORK?

The practitioner chooses appropriate acupressure points and methods of treatment (the use of fingers, thumbs, palms, or elbows) according to the philosophies of Traditional Chinese Medicine, your specific condition, and your medical history. As the practitioner applies pressure to these points, obstructions in the flow of healing energy dissolve, your muscles and ligaments relax, and the body returns to healthier structure. The amount of pressure placed upon a particular point depends on your tolerance of that pressure. A deep, constant circular movement is the primary objective. Treatment time per point can range anywhere from a few seconds to five minutes, or until relief occurs.

The approach of acupressure is very similar to that of acupuncture (see page 16), since both types of treatment are based on the philosophies of Traditional Chinese Medicine. The main difference is that acupressure uses only finger, hand, and elbow pressure—no needles or substances are involved.

## WHAT TO EXPECT

You should expect to be treated in a safe, clean, and comfortable environment. The practitioner will take a full medical history, including examination through observation and questioning. He or she will address all relevant information, characteristics, and symptoms. Next, the acupressurist will check the alignment of your spine. Results from these evaluations will determine the cause of the problem and the areas to be treated.

Acupressure sessions usually take place on a padded treatment table or on a treatment chair. You should wear comfortable clothing that allows for free movement. A treatment gown may have to be worn, depending on the part of body that requires therapeutic attention. The practitioner should be especially sensitive to draping procedures, making sure to expose only the necessary area.

A completed acupressure session will result in effects that are similar to those achieved by a massage, including: increased blood and nutrient circulation; the release of endorphins; and the elimination of waste matter, especially lactic acid, from the muscles. Because acupressure dislodges toxins, you may experience a sensation of lightheadedness, but it will pass quickly. To cleanse the system, it is recommended that you drink plenty of water after a treatment session.

## COST/DURATION

*$60–$90 per session/60 minutes*

Response to acupressure varies according to the condition. Some acute problems, such as headaches and sinusitis, often are relieved after one session. Chronic conditions, such as arthritis, asthma, or sciatica, usually require a number of treatments before the body experiences a significant result.

## CREDENTIALS/EDUCATION

*AOBTA: American Organization for Bodywork Therapies of Asia*

*Diplomate in Asian Bodywork Therapy (NCCAOM): Diplomate in Asian Bodywork Therapy*

*Dipl. A.B.T. (NCCAOM): Diplomate in Asian Bodywork Therapy*

*NCBTMB: National Certification Board for Therapeutic Massage and Bodywork*

There is no state licensing specifically for the practice of acupressure in the United States. However, there are some states that have Massage/Bodywork licensing laws that include Acupressure in that category and accept the National Certification Exam for Therapeutic Massage and Bodywork (NCETMB) as part of its criteria. Further, some of these states also accept the NCCAOM (National Certification Commission for Acupuncture and Oriental Medicine) ABT (Asian Bodywork Therapy) Exam. Since licensing varies from state to state, it is recommended that you seek a practitioner who has graduated from and been certified by an accredited school of acupressure. The members of the organizations that are listed at the conclusion of this section are required to meet certain professional and academic standards. A referral from these organizations will indicate that an individual has received proper training.

Practitioners who are members of the American Organization for Bodywork Therapies of Asia may use AOBTA after their names to denote that they have met the criteria necessary to join this organization. There are two levels of membership. A Certified Practitioner has had a minimum of 500 hours of training. An Associate has a minimum of 150 hours of training. Those practitioners who have passed the ABT exam given by the NCCAOM can use either "Diplomate in Asian Bodywork Therapy (NCCAOM)" or "Dipl. A.B.T. (NCCAOM)". These practitioners have had a minimum of 500 hours of training.

## HOW TO FIND A PRACTITIONER

The best way to find a practitioner of acupressure is to contact the professional organizations listed below to get a referral for an acupressurist in your area, or to a nearby acupressure training institute. Many schools offer training clinics that provide treatments at reduced rates. It is important to note that qualified prac-

titioners of acupressure are not necessarily members of these organizations. Another way to locate an acupressurist is to look in the yellow pages under "acupressure"; "health services"; "holistic/wholistic centers"; and/or "holistic/wholistic practitioners."

## PROFESSIONAL ORGANIZATIONS

American Organization for Bodywork Therapies of Asia
  (AOBTA)
1010 Haddonfield-Berlin Road, Suite 408
Voorhees, NJ 08043-3514
(856) 782-1616
fax: (856) 782-1653
email: aobta@prodigy.net
website: www.aobta.org

National Certification Commission for Acupuncture and
  Oriental Medicine (NCCAOM)
11 Canal Center Plaza, Suite 300
Alexandria, VA 22314
(703) 548-9004
fax: (703) 548-9079
email: info@nccaom.org
website: www.nccaom.org

National Certification Board for Therapeutic Massage
  and Bodywork
8201 Greensboro Drive, Suite 300
McLean, VA 22102
(800) 296-0664 or (703) 610-9015
email: info@ncbtmb.com
website: www.ncbtmb.com

## RECOMMENDED READING

Kenyon, Julian, M.D. *Acupressure Techniques: A Self-Help Guide.* Rochester, VT: Healing Arts Press, 1998.

# ACUPUNCTURE

## WHAT IS IT?

Acupuncture is an ancient Chinese method of healing that involves the insertion of fine needles at specific points on the body. Archaeologists now believe that acupuncture may have been practiced as far back as the Stone Age; needle-like instruments made of jade were discovered at excavation sites near the ancient city of Yin, China. Traditional Chinese Medicine (see page 151) is based on the concept that a universal life energy—*chi*—is present in every living creature. This energy circulates throughout the body along specific pathways, called *meridians*. As long as energy flows freely, health is maintained. If, however, the chi becomes blocked, the system is disrupted and pain and illness result. Acupuncture works to unblock the pathways by stimulating certain points along the meridians.

## CONDITIONS THAT RESPOND BEST

According to the World Health Organization of the United Nations, some of the many conditions for which acupuncture is considered an appropriate treatment are:

- Acne
- Allergies
- Anxiety
- Arthritis
- Asthma
- Back pain
- Bell's palsy
- Bronchitis
- Bursitis
- Cerebral palsy
- Colds and flus
- Colitis
- Constipation
- Deafness
- Depression
- Diabetes
- Diarrhea
- Dizziness
- Earaches
- Eating disorders
- Eczema
- Eyesight problems
- Hay fever
- Headaches
- Hemorrhoids
- Hepatitis

- High blood pressure
- Human immuno-deficiency virus (HIV)
- Hormonal imbalance
- Hypoglycemia
- Impotence
- Indigestion
- Infertility
- Insomnia
- Menstrual irregularities, cramps
- Morning sickness
- Neuralgia
- Pelvic inflammatory disease (PID)
- Polio
- Premenstrual syndrome (PMS)
- Ringing in the ears (tinnitus)
- Sciatica
- Sinus infections
- Sore throats
- Sprains
- Stiff neck
- Stress-related disorders
- Stroke
- Substance abuse
- Temporomandibular joint (TMJ) syndrome
- Tendonitis
- Trigeminal neuralgia
- Ulcers
- Vaginitis

## HOW DOES IT WORK?

Acupuncture stimulates physical reactions in the body, including changes in brain activity, blood chemistry, endocrine functions, blood pressure, heart rate, and immune system response. Medical research shows that acupuncture rouses the body's natural healing abilities to regulate red and white blood cell counts, trigger the production of endorphins, and control blood pressure. These findings begin to explain acupuncture's ability to affect a wide range of illnesses.

The practitioner will diagnose your condition and choose the appropriate acupuncture points according to the concepts of Traditional Chinese Medicine. The acupuncturist primarily uses two techniques: acupuncture and moxibustion.

*Acupuncture,* also called needle therapy, is the insertion of hair-thin, sterile, disposable needles into selected points on the body. When the needle stimulates the acupuncture point, a warm, tingling sensation often is felt. *Moxibustion,* also called heat therapy, involves the burning of a cigar-shaped roll of *moxa*—an herb also known as mugwort, or *Artemisia vulgaris*—above the acupuncture point. Another method includes laying a small slice of fresh ginger root directly on the treatment site, and then placing a piece of dried moxa on top of the ginger. The moxa is ignited, quickly burns on the ginger slice, and the juice from the ginger permeates the aching area. Moxibustion results in a deep penetrating heat and subsequent pain relief. The heat not only has a soothing effect, but also opens the pores of the skin, allowing the healing properties of the ginger to enter the body. Ginger is known for its ability to provide internal warmth. Moxibustion is an extremely effective treatment for conditions of weakness and sensitivity to cold.

The primary focus of acupuncture is to correct the underlying cause of the disease and to produce a lasting cure. Several factors determine the extent to which a person is helped by acupuncture and moxibustion. These include the nature and severity of the health problem, the length of time the problem has existed, and the amount of physical damage caused by the problem. But the most important factor is the strength of each person's recuperative powers, which encompasses a person's age, physical and emotional health, determination, and attitude towards the outcome of treatment.

## WHAT TO EXPECT

You should expect to be treated in a safe, clean, and comfortable environment where privacy and confidentiality are maintained. The practitioner will take a full medical history, including examination through observation and questioning. He or she will address all relevant information, characteristics, and symptoms. Results from this evaluation will determine the cause of the problem and the areas to be treated.

Acupuncture sessions usually take place on a padded treatment table or on a treatment chair. You should wear comfortable clothing that allows for free movement. A treatment gown may have to be worn, depending on the part of the body that requires therapeutic attention. The practitioner should be especially sensitive to draping procedures, making sure to expose only the necessary area.

Many people worry that acupuncture will be painful, but treatments are practically painless. Acupuncture needles are hair-thin, sterile, stainless steel, disposable, and generally cause no bleeding. They are far different from the hypodermic needles used for injections. The skin is cleansed with alcohol before and after treatment. You may feel a minor tingling upon insertion, as the needle reaches the correct point under the skin. Sometimes a slight heat or numbness is experienced, but these sensations are only momentary. In most cases, the needles can hardly be felt at all; often, patients are unaware that insertion is taking place. Once a client has experienced the first session, he or she usually feels happy with the procedure and comfortable with returning for additional acupuncture treatments.

Most people who have been treated by acupuncture notice a considerable improvement in their general health. One of the greatest advantages of this approach is the absence of any harmful side effects associated with its use. Patients sometimes report feeling lightheaded, even euphoric, after treatments. In order to stabilize the body, a few moments of rest after a session is advised.

## COST/DURATION

*$60–$225 per session/approximately 50 minutes*

The number of necessary treatments varies with different conditions; a chronic problem is likely to require a greater number of treatments than an acute problem, which can respond to a single acupuncture session. A series of six to ten treatments is considered typical. Acupuncture is more effective when treatments take place in close proximity to each other, such as having two or three sessions in one week.

## CREDENTIALS/EDUCATION

*C.A.: Certified Acupuncturist*
*Dipl.Ac. (NCCAOM): Diplomate in Acupuncture*
*Diplomate in Acupuncture (NCCAOM): Diplomate in Acupuncture*

*L.Ac.Lic.Ac.: Licensed Acupuncturist*
*M.Ac.: Master of Acupuncture*
*R.Ac.: Registered Acupuncturist*

The regulation of acupuncture practice differs from state to state. While some do not require acupuncture practitioners to graduate from an accredited program, growing numbers of states have instituted this as a prerequisite for state licensure. A non-physician acupuncturist must have more than two years of training at an accredited program, be licensed or registered in your state if applicable, and/or have passed the National Certification Commission for Acupuncture and Oriental Medicine (NCCAOM) exam, which requires at least 1,725 hours of acupuncture training. Safe and effective practice standards have been established by the NCCAOM. All practitioners certified by this commission or by the state comply with strict regulations for proper needle sterilization and handling.

A physician acupuncturist must have at least 200 hours of acupuncture training and should be a member of the American Academy of Medical Acupuncture, which requires proof of training for membership.

## HOW TO FIND A PRACTITIONER

The best way to find an acupuncturist is to contact the professional organizations listed below, which will refer you to practitioners in your area or to a nearby acupuncture training institute. Many schools offer training clinics that provide treatments at reduced rates. It is important to note that qualified acupuncturists are not necessarily members of this organization. Another way to find a practitioner is to look in the yellow pages under "acupuncture"; "health services"; "holistic/wholistic centers"; and/or "holistic /wholistic practitioners."

## PROFESSIONAL ORGANIZATIONS

National Certification Commission for Acupuncture and
    Oriental Medicine (NCCAOM)
11 Canal Center Plaza, Suite 300
Alexandria, VA 22314

(703) 548-9004
fax: (703) 548-9079
email: info@nccaom.org
website: www.nccaom.org

Acupuncture and Oriental Medicine Alliance (AOMA)
6405 43rd Avenue Ct. NW, Suite B
Gig Harbor, WA 98335
(253) 851-6896
fax: (253) 851-6883
website: www.aomalliance.org

## RECOMMENDED READING

Firebrace, Peter, and Sandra Hill. *Acupuncture: How It Works, How It Cures.* New Canaan, CT: Keats Publishing, 1994.

Williams, Tom. *Chinese Medicine.* Rockport, MA: Element Books, 1997.

# THE ALEXANDER TECHNIQUE

## WHAT IS IT?

The Alexander Technique is an educational process that endeavors to identify poor postural habits and replace them with better body mechanics. The main objective is to develop conscious control of your movements in all activities. This technique was developed in the nineteenth century by an Australian actor, Frederick Mathias Alexander (1869–1956), who suffered from chronic hoarseness when performing. Discouraged by medical treatments and vocal studies that could not give him more than temporary relief, he took matters into his own hands. Setting up a three-way mirror, Alexander determined to closely analyze his body movements as he practiced his Shakespeare. He found that while some of his postures were right for the characters, they were not right for his voice muscles. Alexander noticed how he pressed his head down onto the back of his neck and compressed his spine. This produced tension throughout his body, which resulted in his hoarseness. The actor realized that by consciously holding his head so that it did not put pressure on the back of his neck, he was able to move more freely and efficiently. Alexander continued to observe himself, correcting old habits whenever they returned. With time, his sensory perception improved to such a degree that he was able to feel his inappropriate posture without having to watch himself in the mirror. Alexander perfected his technique over nine years of self-study. He began working with others, writing extensively about the technique, and training instructors in Australia, Great Britain, and the United States.

## CONDITIONS THAT RESPOND BEST

The Alexander Technique is a helpful option for the treatment of many conditions that result from poor posture, including:

- Anxiety
- Arthritis
- Backache
- Balance, coordination difficulties
- Breathing disorders
- Bursitis
- Circulatory disorders
- Disc problems
- Eye, ear, nose, throat problems
- Headaches
- Muscular tics, cramps
- Neck, shoulder stiffness
- Pinched nerves
- Rheumatism
- Round shoulders
- Sciatica
- Speech problems
- Stress-related disorders
- Temporomandibular joint (TMJ) syndrome
- Tennis elbow
- Tension
- Ulcers
- Whiplash

## HOW DOES IT WORK?

Poor postural habits and unhealthy body mechanics, such as slouching in a chair or lifting objects without bending the knees, can lead to aches, pains, muscle tightness, and the inability of the body to function properly. The Alexander Technique works toward correcting these bad habits. The instructor teaches simple exercises designed to improve balance, posture, and coordination. He or she also offers gentle hands-on guidance and verbal instruction to train you in the optimal use of your body. Benefits of this approach include a release of excess tension in the body and a lengthening of the spine. As a result, you will experience greater freedom and flexibility in movement, as well as improved posture, appearance, and general health. Upon completion of training, you should be able to correct yourself immediately when destructive habits return.

## WHAT TO EXPECT

Expect a comfortable, professional office where privacy and confidentiality are maintained. Before beginning instruction, the practitioner will conduct an examination through observation and questioning. He or she will observe your posture and body mechanics during various activities, and then will focus on specific movements. The lesson may center around something as basic as getting up from a chair. You should wear comfortable clothing that allows for free movement.

The instructor applies his or her knowledge of proper technique and directs you carefully. As mentioned above, hands-on guidance and verbal coaching are part of the session. The process is painless; there are no needles, mechanical devices, or oils used.

## COST/DURATION

*$50–$85 per session/30–50 minutes*

The necessary number of sessions depends on your motivation and on the severity of the physical condition; the average number is thirty. The frequency of sessions, or how often they occur within a given time period, varies considerably.

## CREDENTIALS/EDUCATION

*AmSAT: American Society of the Alexander Technique*

An instructor of the Alexander Technique must be certified by the American Society of the Alexander Technique (AmSAT). This credential indicates that the instructor has completed a three-year, 1,600-hour training program at an approved school. In addition, professionals can become a board-certified Alexander Technique teacher by meeting additional requirements and peer review.

## HOW TO FIND A PRACTITIONER

The best way to find a practitioner of the Alexander Technique is to contact the professional organization listed below, which will provide information on instructors in your area. Another method is to look in the yellow pages under "Alexander Technique"; "health services"; "holistic/wholistic centers"; and/or "holistic/wholistic practitioners."

## PROFESSIONAL ORGANIZATION

American Society of the Alexander Technique (AmSAT)
P.O. Box 60008
Florence, MA 01062
(800) 473-0620
fax: (413) 584-3097
website: www.alexandertech.org

## RECOMMENDED READING

MacDonald, Glynn. *Illustrated Elements of Alexander Technique.* Hammersmith, London: Element, 2002.

Gelb, Michael. *Body Learning: An Introduction to the Alexander Technique.* New York: H. Holt and Co., 1996.

# AQUATIC THERAPY

## WHAT IS IT?

Water is an ideal environment in which to promote healing. Aquatic therapy, also known as water therapy, has been used for centuries to invigorate the body and relieve pain. The exercise, stretching, and relaxation techniques take place in a warm, shallow pool that is specifically designed for therapeutic purposes.

Gentle and rhythmic movements are performed from seated, standing, walking, and/or floating positions. In addition to targeting problem areas, the stretching and conditioning activities are designed to benefit all major muscle groups.

## CONDITIONS THAT RESPOND BEST

Aquatic therapy is appropriate for the treatment of a variety of conditions, including:

- Anxiety
- Arthritis
- Back pain
- Balance problems
- Chronic orthopedic problems
- Chronic pain
- Hypertension
- Incapacity to perform traditional exercise programs
- Inflammation
- Muscle pain
- Neurological injuries
- Obesity
- Orthopedic injuries
- Respiratory problems

Aquatic therapy also promotes the achievement of the following exercise goals:
- Aerobic conditioning
- Enhancement of flexibility, endurance, and strength

## HOW DOES IT WORK?

Many aquatic therapy facilities are equipped with a heated pool (92°F to 99°F), as well as an additional pool containing cooler water. The warm water stimulates and then relaxes tired, aching muscles. By calming the nerves and increasing circulation, this therapy decreases muscle stiffness. The cooler, more invigorating water helps reduce muscle swelling and pain by constricting the blood vessels. Patients with non-weight-bearing injuries and those who cannot tolerate traditional exercise programs find the buoyancy of water to be the perfect medium in which to accelerate the healing process.

The goal of aquatic therapy is to develop freer body movements that increase strength, flexibility, and endurance. You begin with guidance from the instructor and gradually learn to manage your own therapy program. This approach encourages you to participate in, and take responsibility for, your own recovery.

## WHAT TO EXPECT

Your full medical history will be taken before therapy begins; special attention will be given to conditions that hot or cold temperatures might aggravate or worsen. Then you will enter the pool area, which should be clean and well-maintained. The pool water should be clear and at the proper temperature. A bathing suit is necessary, as well as a warm robe to be worn after exiting the pool. Be aware that you do not need to know how to swim. The instructor will guide the class through exercise, stretching, and relaxation techniques. Participants generally wear an aquatic belt (a non-restrictive flotation device). Other aquatic resistance equipment may be used during the exercise session.

In a special type of aquatic therapy called WATSU (water shiatsu), the shiatsu practitioner applies shiatsu massage techniques in chest-high, warm water. He or she will guide you through a series of slow, flowing movements that aim at releasing tension and decreasing pain. Because the instructor supplies much of the support in the water, the contact is more extensive than standard aquatic therapy and may not appeal to everyone. (For more information on shiatsu, see page 131.)

## COST/DURATION

*$10–$45 per class/30–60 minutes*
*$60–$120 per individual training*

You should expect to commit to a series of six to eight aquatic therapy sessions for maximum benefit.

## CREDENTIALS/EDUCATION

*Certified Aquatic Exercise Instructor*
*CPR and First Aid certification*
*W.S.I.: Water Safety Instructor (Red Cross certification)*

Although there are no mandatory requirements or state regulations for aquatic therapists, it is recommended that you select a

# *Hydrotherapy*

The therapeutic use of water dates back to ancient Greek and Roman times; it has been used for centuries to promote healing and to maintain good health. *Hydrotherapy* is the application of water in its various forms (liquid, solid, and vapor) for health treatment purposes. This approach is often used as an adjunct treatment to many alternative medicine approaches, particularly massage (see page 87), and to conventional medical programs such as physical therapy and nursing care.

The various applications of hot and cold water treatments create different physiological effects on the body. These effects can be either stimulating or sedating to the nervous and circulatory systems. For example, short applications of cold can have a stimulating effect, while longer applications of cold can have a sedating effect. The application of heat generally relaxes the body. Prolonged treatments of extremely hot or cold temperatures should be applied under close supervision or avoided.

Hydrotherapy offers many different treatment options, some of which are:

- hot/cold packs
- hot tubs
- ice massage
- Jacuzzis
- moist heat packs
- saunas
- sitz baths
- steam baths
- whirlpools

Both hydrotherapy and aquatic therapy rely on the natural healing effects of water. Hydrotherapy differs from aquatic therapy in that the client *passively* receives the water-based treatment; unlike aquatic therapy, there is no exercise routine involved.

practitioner who has been certified. The level of certifications will vary, depending on the facility where the classes take place. Hospital-based programs generally have higher credential requirements. Many facilities that employ physical therapists and occupational therapists provide aquatic therapy. YMCAs, YWCAs, and health and fitness centers are also likely to offer aquatic therapy programs. The professional organization listed below also certifies aquatic exercise instructors in various courses.

## HOW TO FIND A PRACTITIONER

The best way to locate an aquatic therapist is to contact the professional organizations listed below, which will refer you to instructors in your area. Another method is to look in the yellow pages under "aquatic therapy"; "fitness facilities"; "health clubs"; "health services"; "holistic/wholistic centers"; "holistic/wholistic practitioners"; "hydrotherapy"; "physical therapy centers"; "YMCA/YWCA"; and/or the local chapter of the American Red Cross.

## PROFESSIONAL ORGANIZATION

Aquatic Exercise Association
3439 Technology Drive, Unit 6
Nokomis, FL 34274-3627
(941) 486-8600 or (888) AEA-WAVE/(888) 232-9283
fax: (941) 486-8820
email: info@aeawave.com
website: www.aeawave.com

Red Cross (local chapters found in your yellow pages)

## RECOMMENDED READING

Huey, Lynda, and Robert Forster, PT. *The Complete Waterpower Workout Book.* New York: Random House, 1993.

# AROMATHERAPY

## WHAT IS IT?

The power of aroma is evident through its capacity to affect the emotions and the body. For example, the scent of a rose can stimulate feelings of happiness and euphoria. The fragrances of lavender and chamomile are helpful in combating insomnia. Aromatherapy is an approach that obtains aromatic, essential oils from herbs and flowers and assigns them as therapeutic treatments.

Aromatherapy dates back thousands of years. The term *aromatherapy* was first established when French chemist René Maurice Gattefosse published his work, *Aromatherapie,* in 1937. (Years earlier, Gattefosse had experimented with the use of essential oils to treat wounds. He personally experienced the healing properties of lavender when he applied it to burns on his own hands.) In the 1950s, Marguerite Maury, a French woman whose husband was a homeopathic doctor, researched essential oils for medical and cosmetic applications. Aromatherapy was eventually brought to Great Britain through the work of massage therapists and estheticians. Since then, its practice has grown extensively.

## CONDITIONS THAT RESPOND BEST

Aromatherapy can improve general health and relieve/reduce a number of specific conditions, including:

- Anxiety
- Arthritis
- Asthma
- Back problems
- Bronchitis
- Bruises
- Colds, coughs, sore throats
- Colic
- Constipation
- Depression
- Eating disorders
- Eye, ear, nose, throat problems
- Fatigue
- Headaches
- Hemorrhoids
- Hormonal imbalance
- Indigestion
- Insomnia
- Low blood pressure
- Motion sickness
- Muscle strain
- Nausea
- Pain
- Poor circulation
- Premenstrual syndrome (PMS)
- Rheumatism
- Sinusitis
- Skin conditions
- Sunburn
- Varicose veins
- Water retention

This approach also can contribute to the achievement of the following health goals:

- Enhancement of mood
- Increase in vitality
- Relaxation

## HOW DOES IT WORK?

Your sense of smell is connected to the part of your brain that controls the autonomic (involuntary) nervous system. As a result, you respond immediately and involuntarily to scent. The powerful perfume of the essential oils stimulates the release of neurotransmitters in your brain. These brain chemicals can have effects that are calming, sedating, pain-reducing, stimulating, or euphoric. In addition, when essential oils are applied to the skin in specially prepared lotions, they can serve as antibacterial, anti-inflammatory, and astringency agents. Each essential oil is known for its aroma and characteristic therapeutic effects.

The essential oils used for aromatherapy are derived through a steam-distillation process. Plant materials are heated in water, resulting in the release of oils in the form of vapors. These vapors, as well as the steam from the water, then move through a cooling tube in which they are converted back to liquid form. From this liquid, the concentrated essential oil is gathered, along with a less concentrated solution of plant water, called *hydrosol*. Both of these substances are used in aromatherapy. The oils and hydrosols produce therapeutic effects on the mind, emotions, and respiration through several methods of inhalation: placing drops of oil on a handkerchief or in steaming hot water; using a diffuser—a device that, when heated, spreads the vapors throughout a room; spritzing hydrosols from a spray bottle into the air or on the face; and soaking in therapeutic baths, which utilizes both inhalation and absorption.

When diluted in prepared lotions, oils can be applied directly to the skin. The aromatherapist generally uses such lotions during massage treatments. (For information on massage, see page 87.) This method allows you to benefit not only from the aroma, but also from the absorption of the oils into the skin. Practitioners believe that these oils are carried throughout the body via the bloodstream, and can strengthen and heal muscle tissue, joints, and organs.

## WHAT TO EXPECT

You should expect to be treated in a safe and clean environment. The aromatherapist will begin with a full investigation into your medical history, including examination through observation and questioning. All relevant information, characteristics, and symptoms will be addressed. Next, he or she will blend an appropriate oil to be used during treatment. Aromatherapy massage usually takes place on a padded treatment table or in a treatment chair. You should wear comfortable clothing that allows for free movement. A treatment gown may have to be worn, depending on the part of the body that requires therapeutic attention. The practitioner should be especially sensitive to draping procedures, making sure to expose only the necessary area. This approach should promote relaxation and increase your sense of well-being. Often, you will have the opportunity to purchase the remainder of the oil for at-home use.

You can conduct your own aromatherapy through methods of inhalation, including the use of diffusers, spray bottles, and therapeutic baths. At-home therapy can be safe and effective, but caution is required. Essential oils are very potent due to their high concentrations; each oil has its own benefits and hazards. It is recommended that you read an aromatherapy resource book, take a course, or visit a qualified aromatherapist before experimenting with the oils. Hydrosols are extremely gentle and are practically free of irritants. They can be used more liberally, particularly in atomizers.

## COST/DURATION

*Individual: $60–$80 per session/60 minutes*
*Informational class: $30/60–120 minutes*

If you wish to take home any remaining oil after a treatment session, you may be expected to pay an additional fee.

## CREDENTIALS/EDUCATION

*NAHA: National Association for Holistic Aromatherapy*
*RA™: Registered Aromatherapist*

There are currently no licensing procedures or accrediting boards for the practice of aromatherapy in the United States. The National Association for Holistic Aromatherapy (NAHA) has set up guidelines and offers a listing of schools that adhere to these standards. A Level Two course at one of these schools leads to certification in aromatherapy. Additionally, there is a national exam offered by the Aromatherapy Registration Council (ARC). Passing of the exam allows the use of the credential RA™, registered aromatherapist. Aromatherapy is primarily practiced by massage therapists. However, other healthcare providers also incorporate aromatherapy into their practices. It is recommended that you seek a practitioner who, in addition to having credentials in his or her specific field, has additional training in aromatherapy.

## HOW TO FIND A PRACTITIONER

The best way to find a practitioner of aromatherapy is to contact the professional organizations listed below, which will refer you to an aromatherapist in your area or to a local aromatherapy school. It is important to note that practitioners of aromatherapy are not necessarily members of these professional organizations. Another way to locate an aromatherapist is to look in the yellow pages under "aromatherapy"; "health services"; "holistic/wholistic centers"; "holistic/wholistic practitioners"; "massage"; and/or "therapeutic massage."

## PROFESSIONAL ORGANIZATIONS

National Association for Holistic Aromatherapy (NAHA)
4509 Interlake Avenue N., #233
Seattle, WA 98103-6773
(888) ASK-NAHA / (888) 275-6242 or (206) 547-2164
fax: (206) 547-2680
email: info@naha.org
website: www.naha.org

Aromatherapy Registration Council (ARC)
email: info@aromatherapycouncil.org

website: www.aromatherapycouncil.org (you can download
a register of Registered Aromatherapists™)

## RECOMMENDED READING

Maxwell-Hudson, Clare. *Aromatherapy Massage.* New York: DK
Publishing, Inc., 1997.

Wilson, Roberta. *Aromatherapy for Vibrant Health and Beauty: A
Practical A to Z Reference to Aromatherapy Treatments for Health,
Skin, and Hair Problems Using Essential Oils.* Garden City Park, NY:
Avery Publishing Group, 1995.

# AYURVEDA

## WHAT IS IT?

Ayurveda is a natural healthcare system that was developed in
India over 5,000 years ago. It teaches individuals to become active
participants in the maintenance of their body systems, focusing
on how to prevent disease and teaching methods of returning
to good health. Ayurvedic medicine achieves these goals by
combining various approaches, such as exercise (gentle yoga
positions, see page 62, and brisk, half-hour daily walks); herbal
remedies (*rasayana* are special herbs and minerals used to promote longevity, see also page 66); massage (see page 87); meditation (progressive relaxation and deep breathing, see page 119);
and nutritional counseling (see page 92). Deepak Chopra, a physician from India who came to the United States in 1970, has popularized Ayurvedic practice and philosophy through numerous
books, tapes, and lectures. Through his work and the dedicated
efforts of many alternative healthcare professionals, numerous
people are learning to trust and develop their own powers of
mind and body.

## CONDITIONS THAT RESPOND BEST

Ayurvedic medicine benefits any individual who is interested in promoting optimal health. It is also appropriate in the treatment of a wide range of physical and emotional illnesses. Just a few of the many conditions that respond to Ayurveda are:

- Allergies
- Back pain
- Balance, coordination disorders
- Cardiovascular disorders
- Circulatory disorders
- Dermatological conditions
- Digestive disorders
- Eating disorders
- Emotional health disorders (including stress, anxiety)
- Endocrine disorders
- Eye, ear, nose, throat disorders
- Immune disorders
- Musculoskeletal disorders
- Nervous system disorders
- Reproductive disorders
- Respiratory disorders
- Substance abuse
- Teeth, jaw conditions

## HOW DOES IT WORK?

Ayurveda works through a process of identification and education. The practitioner asks questions about your present lifestyle; eating and sleeping habits; emotional and physical makeup; and food and environmental preferences. Ayurvedic medicine follows two chief principles. First, your mind has a profound influence on your physical body; a pattern of negative thoughts will ultimately create illness, while positive thoughts will help return the body to good health. Becoming aware of your mind's role in maintaining or destroying health is an integral part of healing through Ayurveda.

The second principle of Ayurvedic medicine maintains that each person is born with a specific makeup or body type. The term used for body type is *prakriti*, a Sanskrit word meaning "nature." There are three general body types which are explained below. Your constitution, as described through your given body type, is of prime importance to this approach. Treatment is designed according to prakriti.

Ayurvedic philosophy holds that the body has three basic operating principles, called *doshas*, which are needed for healthy functioning. The *vata* dosha is responsible for respiration, blood circulation, digestion, and nervous system functioning. The *pitta* dosha conducts the processing of nutrients, air, and water in the body. Finally, the *kapha* dosha manages the structure of the body and includes muscles, fat, and bones. Body type—prakriti—is assigned according to which dosha is most prominent in a person's system. Thus, you will be labeled as a vata, pitta, or kapha, although some body types are a combination of two of these systems. Certain characteristics are attributed to each prakriti, a few of which are as follows: the vata tends to be slim, nervous, very energetic, and erratic in both behavior and body systems; the pitta is generally of medium size, fervent, and intelligent, with a strict regularity of mind and body; the kapha often has a heavy build, slow-functioning systems, and a relaxed nature that expresses both sympathy and stubbornness.

Using your prakriti as a guide, the Ayurvedic practitioner can determine exactly what is good for you and what is not, including types of foods, exercise, medical treatments, environmental surroundings, and career choices. Deviation from or lack of attention to this plan can create an imbalance that results in future illness. Your treatment program will be designed to bring the three doshas into harmonious balance. The goal of Ayurveda is not to identify disease, but to help an individual achieve a lifestyle that will ultimately balance body and mind for optimum health. Meditation, herbal remedies, and/or massage may be suggested, with referrals made to individual practitioners in these specialties. *Marma therapy*, a form of self-massage, is often recommended and can be taught by a practitioner of this specialty.

As mentioned previously, Ayurvedic medicine will educate you on how the environment in which you live and work influences your state of health. Many people thrive on the hustle and bustle of city life; they enjoy the crowds and desire to be a part of the action. Others prefer the serenity of living in the suburbs, away from crowded city streets. Often, people are faced with the challenge of working or living in an environment to which they do not adapt easily. Individuals who are most comfortable in quiet environments may find themselves working in high-stress, chaotic settings. In order to remain physically and emotionally healthy, it is important for such people to re-energize, using stress-reducing techniques that are taught through Ayurvedic exercises and meditation. If you find yourself straining against the surroundings in which you spend most of your day, your practitioner will give you advice on how to cope with the tensions and how to restore yourself to health.

## WHAT TO EXPECT

You should expect a comfortable, professional environment where privacy and confidentiality are maintained. The first visit is generally a consultation at which a full medical history is taken. The practitioner will ask you questions that identify who you are, rather than what disease you have. He or she will address all relevant information, characteristics, and symptoms. Results from this evaluation determine the cause of health problems and a treatment plan.

The Ayurvedic practitioner will discuss your body type and make recommendations pertaining to diet, exercise, meditation, massage, and medical treatments. He or she will offer referrals to specialists of the recommended approaches. Again, the process of Ayurvedic medicine involves identification and education. You will be encouraged to maintain your own health as much as possible, and will be guided on a path of daily health awareness.

## COST/DURATION

*Initial Visit: $90–$225/60–180 minutes*
*Follow-up Visit: $60–$90/30–60 minutes*

During the initial consultation, you will receive basic lifestyle information—dietary guidelines, exercise agendas, and suggested environmental changes—that can be applied immediately. Additional specialty treatments will be at extra cost. The overall duration of treatments depends on your specific needs. Keep in mind that you can gain valuable information on Ayurvedic philosophy and practice through informational books, tapes, and videos.

## CREDENTIALS/EDUCATION

*B.A.M.S.: Bachelor of Ayurveda Medical Studies*

There are currently no licensing procedures or accrediting boards concerning the practice of Ayurvedic medicine in the United States. Graduates of courses in Ayurveda can consult with clients, but cannot practice as medical doctors. Some physicians have studied Ayurveda, and many healthcare providers incorporate its philosophies into their current practices. It is recommended that you seek a practitioner who has completed his or her full medical degree in India and holds a B.A.M.S. (Bachelor of Ayurveda Medical Studies). Also, some healthcare practitioners have completed a one-year certificate program and are very capable of consulting on Ayurvedic principles.

## HOW TO FIND A PRACTITIONER

There is no professional organization that offers membership to Ayurveda practitioners. However, the below-listed institute can provide the names of appropriate professionals in your area. Another way to find a practitioner is to look in the yellow pages under "Ayurveda"; "health services"; "holistic/wholistic centers"; and/or "holistic/wholistic practitioners."

## PROFESSIONAL ORGANIZATION

The Ayurvedic Institute
P.O. Box 23445
Albuquerque, NM 87192-1445
(505) 291-9698
fax: (505) 294-7572
website: www.ayurveda.com

## RECOMMENDED READING

Lad, Vasant, B.A.M.S. *The Complete Book of Ayurvedic Home Remedies*. New York: Three Rivers Press, 1998.

# BIOFEEDBACK

## WHAT IS IT?

Being evaluated by biofeedback techniques is like taking a relaxation detector test. Biofeedback uses a simple electronic monitoring device, which is connected by electrodes to the skin's surface, to collect information on vital body functions such as heart rate, blood pressure, muscle tension, brain wave activity, and skin temperature. The practitioner assesses the feedback and teaches the client appropriate relaxation, meditation, and visualization techniques. (For information on relaxation/meditation, refer to page 119.) The client learns to control his or her body's responses and gains consequent health improvement. Ultimately, biofeedback enables a person to gain psychological control over physiological processes.

Studies concerning the mental control of biological conditions began gaining attention in the 1950s, due to the work of Neal E. Miller and several other psychologists. Research was done mostly with animals, sometimes with humans, and continued into the 1960s. Miller's work demonstrated that rats could be taught to control physiological processes such as digestion, blood flow, and heart rate. Such conclusions sparked researchers in the United States to begin looking at the relaxed state of meditating yogis. They studied how such levels of consciousness could be scientifically measured using brain wave biofeedback. Interest in other applications of biofeedback grew rapidly from this point. Today, biofeedback techniques track numerous physiological systems and enable the client to become more conscious of the body's functioning.

## CONDITIONS THAT RESPOND BEST

Biofeedback is an appropriate treatment option for any physical or emotional illness that could benefit from improved relaxation skills. Among the many conditions that respond to biofeedback therapy are:

- Anxiety
- Asthma
- Headaches, migraines
- High blood pressure
- Muscular dysfunction
- Pain
- Stress-related disorders

## HOW DOES IT WORK?

During a biofeedback session, information on a specific body system travels through electrodes that adhere to the skin. This data registers within the biofeedback machine and is changed into signals. These signals can be heard as sounds (beeps), seen as video images (flashes), or monitored by dial readings. They act as feedback, helping you to become more aware of changes in your body. The practitioner instructs you to alter or slow down the signals through the use of relaxation, meditation, and/or visualization. Deep breathing exercises and focusing on positive images may be used.

Because the feedback is immediate, you can work on and improve your relaxation skills from the very first session. The goal is to maintain the acquired skills of relaxation even when the biofeedback device is no longer used. With practice, a healthier physical and emotional state becomes natural.

## WHAT TO EXPECT

You should expect a comfortable, professional office where privacy and confidentiality are maintained. The practitioner will take a full medical history, including examination through observation and questioning, and will address all relevant information, characteristics, and symptoms. During the session, you will be seated near the biofeedback machine. The machine's electrode sensors (wires) will be placed on the surface of your skin, generally on the forehead, neck, back, and/or forefinger. The process is painless. As vital body functions are monitored, the practitioner will guide you through progressive relaxation, meditation, and/or visualization. If the body responds in a healthy manner, readings indicate relaxed muscles, lowered heart rate, or lowered temperature. As practice during and outside the session continues, you will learn to control your body's responses and eventually maintain a relaxed, healthier state without the biofeedback machine.

## COST/DURATION

*$50–$150 per session/50 minutes*

The cost of a treatment session varies according to the education and credentials of the practitioner. The number of treatments needed will depend on the severity of the condition and on your response.

## CREDENTIALS/EDUCATION

*B.C.I.A.C.: Biofeedback Certification Institute of America Certified*

There is no state licensing for biofeedback practitioners. Various healthcare professionals incorporate biofeedback into their practices, including psychiatrists; psychologists; social workers; nurses; physical therapists; occupational therapists; speech therapists; respiratory therapists; exercise physiologists; chiropractors; dentists; and physician's assistants. It is recommended that you seek a healthcare practitioner who has been certified through the Biofeedback Certification Institute of America. This institute sets clear standards and requires a minimum of a bachelor's degree in a health-related area before a candidate can seek certification.

## HOW TO FIND A PRACTITIONER

The best way to find a biofeedback practitioner is to contact the professional organizations listed below, which will refer you to practitioners in your area. Another method is to look in the yellow pages under "biofeedback therapists"; "physicians/psychiatrists"; "psychologists"; and/or "psychotherapists." Also check under "exercise physiologists"; "occupational therapists"; "physical therapists"; and/or "speech therapists," all of whom may use biofeedback in their practices. Local hospitals and medical clinics offer biofeedback services, as well.

## PROFESSIONAL ORGANIZATIONS

Biofeedback Certification Institute of America (BCIA)
10200 W. 44th Avenue, Suite 310
Wheat Ridge, CO 80033-2840
(303) 420-2902

fax: (303) 422-8894
email: bcia@resourcenter.com
website: www.bcia.org

Association for Applied Psychophysiology and Biofeedback
    (AAPB)
10200 W. 44th Avenue, Suite 304
Wheat Ridge, CO 80033-2840
(303) 422-8436
fax: (303) 422-8894
email: aapb@resourcenter.com
website: www.aapb.org

*The AAPB does not certify practitioners, it is geared towards
    research in the field.

## RECOMMENDED READING

Wise, Anna. *The High-Performance Mind: Mastering Brainwaves
for Insight, Healing, and Creativity.* New York: Jeremy P. Tarcher,
1995.

# BODYWORK

*Bodywork* is a general term referring to approaches that use
hands-on techniques to manipulate and balance the musculoskeletal system. Such approaches facilitate healing, increase
energy, relieve pain, and promote relaxation and well-being. The
bodywork therapies discussed in this book are: *acupressure* (see
page 11); *the Alexander Technique* (see page 21); *chiropractic* (see
page 42); *CranioSacral Therapy* (see page 46); *the Feldenkrais Method*
(see page 51); *foot reflexology* (see page 59); *lymphatic massage* (see
page 84); *Rolfing* (see page 127); *shiatsu* (see page 131); *sports
massage* (see page 135); *Swedish massage* (see page 140); *the Trager
approach* (see page 156); and *trigger point therapy* (see page 159).
Please see these individual approach sections for more information.

# CHIROPRACTIC

## WHAT IS IT?

The chiropractic system is based on the belief that a strong, agile, and aligned spine is the key to good health. Trauma or poor posture can result in pressure on the spinal cord, leading to illness and diminished or painful movement. The chiropractor manipulates and makes adjustments to the spine. With the backbone in its proper position, the nervous system is free to send out the necessary signals for the human body to function normally. A chiropractic treatment session might also include dietary advice and nutritional counseling (see page 92), rehabilitative exercises, and advice on job-related body mechanics. Prescription drugs and surgery are not part of chiropractic procedure.

Chiropractic treatment has its origins in ancient China and ancient Greece. Many other civilizations also have incorporated therapeutic spinal manipulations into their healing arts, including the North American Indians, who used a technique that involved walking on the back of the person being treated. In Europe, up until and including the nineteenth century, manipulation was practiced by healers called *bonesetters*. The art of bonesetting was learned and passed down through family lines.

Even though it has been used for centuries, spinal manipulation was not organized into a precise medical science until 1895. That year, Daniel David Palmer, a grocer and teacher from Canada who studied the ancient principles of manipulation, founded the first school of chiropractic training. His son, Bartlett Joshua Palmer, was one of the first graduates of the Palmer Infirmary and Chiropractic Institute in Davenport, Iowa. B.J. Palmer is credited with saving chiropractic care from extinction by preserving many of the original principles established by his father. Today, chiropractic is a booming field that has gained the trust of enormous numbers of clients.

## CONDITIONS THAT RESPOND BEST

Chiropractic is an appropriate therapy for the treatment of many conditions, including:

- Allergies
- Ankle swelling
- Arm, shoulder pain
- Arthritis
- Asthma
- Back pain
- Bronchial conditions
- Bursitis
- Chest pain
- Chronic cough
- Circulation problems
- Colitis
- Constipation
- Diarrhea
- Disc problems
- Diverticulitis
- Dizziness
- Ear, eye problems
- Emphysema
- Fatigue
- Gall bladder problems
- Headaches
- Hemorrhoids
- High blood pressure
- Indigestion
- Insomnia
- Joint pain
- Kidney disorders
- Knee pain
- Leg cramps
- Liver disorders
- Low blood pressure
- Neuralgia
- Prostate disorders
- Rheumatism
- Sciatica
- Shingles
- Sinus trouble
- Sports injuries
- Stiff neck
- Thyroid conditions
- Ulcers
- Whiplash

## HOW DOES IT WORK?

According to chiropractic philosophy, the alignment of the spine is essential for the optimal functioning of the nervous system. The human spine consists of twenty-four bones called *vertebrae*. Discs of cartilage between each pair of vertebrae provide protective cushioning. The spinal cord, which is part of the central nervous system, suspends from the brain and runs through the hollow tunnel of the spine. Small nerve trunks branch off the spinal cord and lead through channels in the vertebrae. When the notches in the vertebrae are aligned correctly, nerves can pass through and function properly. But if the notches are misaligned, the channel distorts and the nerves become entrapped, compressed, or pinched. Dysfunction results, which lowers resistance to infection and disease in the areas of the body that are served by those nerves. The chiropractor's objective is to identify and correct the misalignments through spinal manipulation or adjustment. Additionally, since the back muscles are attached to the spine and give support to the structure, he or she may also integrate muscle work that uses various massage therapy techniques to alleviate tension and/or spasm.

Manipulations are performed by hand, although some chiropractic doctors may use special treatment tables to facilitate the outcome. One example is a table equipped with two rollers; as you lie on your back, the rollers move along your spine, creating a gentle massage and helping the spine to loosen and realign. Chiropractic adjustments can then continue with less pressure. Certain treatment processes also include the application of heat, cold, or ultrasound for muscle relaxation. In addition, chiropractors may offer advice on nutrition and exercise to support the benefits gained from manipulation and to help prevent future problems.

## WHAT TO EXPECT

You should expect a comfortable, professional office where privacy and confidentiality are maintained. During the first visit, your complete medical history will be taken. This makes it possible to ascertain any conditions that might require special precautions. The chiropractor will also examine your spine through touch and/or palpation, looking for problems, irregularities, tenderness, and swelling. Depending upon what is found and the nature of the complaint, the practitioner may feel that x-rays of the spine are necessary. Then the doctor will offer a brief summary of the diagnosed disorder and its extent, reviewing your physical examination and spinal analysis. If appropriate, he or she will suggest prevention techniques relating to the occupational activities and daily habits that might be harming you. Your chiropractor should also discuss the anticipated number of treatments necessary to attain the desired goal.

To begin a chiropractic adjustment, you will lie on a padded treatment table. The chiropractor will assess your back with his or her hands, and then begin manipulation. As adjustment takes place, you might feel a slight snap that is similar to cracking your knuckles. Some discomfort may occur, but it should not be intense. Chiropractic, if conducted properly, will not be painful. In fact, you may experience a subtle easing of pain and an improvement in the ability to move your body.

## COST/DURATION

*Initial Visit: $60–$225 (depending on diagnostic testing)/30–60 minutes*
*Follow-up Visit: $30–$75/10–20 minutes*

The range for all treatments is two to fifteen visits, varying according to the severity of the condition. Many chiropractic doctors offer free consultation.

## CREDENTIALS/EDUCATION

*D.C.: Doctor of Chiropractic*

All states require chiropractors to be licensed. They must graduate from an accredited college of chiropractic to earn the degree of Doctor of Chiropractic (D.C.), then pass an examination from the National Board of Chiropractic Examiners, as well as a state board exam. To maintain licensure, chiropractors are required to fulfill continuing education hours each year.

## HOW TO FIND A PRACTITIONER

The best way to find a chiropractor is to contact the professional organization listed below, which will refer you to a practitioner in your area. Another option is to look in the yellow pages under "chiropractors."

## PROFESSIONAL ORGANIZATION

American Chiropractic Association (ACA)

1701 Clarendon Boulevard
Arlington, VA 22209
(800) 986-4636
fax: (703) 243-2593
website: www.amerchiro.org

## RECOMMENDED READING

Gandee, William S., D.C., and Peggy Russell. *Triumph Over Illness: What You Should Know About the Power of Chiropractic Care.* Garden City Park, NY: Avery Publishing Group, 1997.

McGill, Leonard. *The Chiropractor's Health Book: Simple, Natural Exercises for Relieving Headaches, Tension and Back Pain.* New York: Crown Publishing, 1997.

Wilk, Chester A., D.C. *Medicine, Monopolies, and Malice: How the Medical Establishment Tried to Destroy Chiropractic in the U.S.* Garden City Park, NY: Avery Publishing Group, 1996.

# CRANIOSACRAL THERAPY

## WHAT IS IT?

The craniosacral system includes the bones of the cranium (skull, face, and mouth), the spine and sacrum (the lower end of the spine), the membranes that connect the cranium to the sacrum, and the cerebrospinal fluid. CranioSacral Therapy uses gentle hands-on techniques to treat stress and restriction in this region, helping to create a healthier environment for proper central nervous system functioning. This approach involves applied pressure that never exceeds the weight of a nickel. Practitioners can detect and correct craniosacral imbalances, resulting in general health enhancement for the treated individual.

CranioSacral Therapy has its origins in the work of William Garner Sutherland (1873-1954). In the early 1900s, as a student at the American School of Osteopathy in Kirksville, Missouri,

Sutherland began questioning whether the bones of the adult skull were moveable. He researched his idea over the next twenty years, using helmet-like devices that applied pressure to different parts of his skull. He documented his own physical and emotional reactions to this compression, and concluded the existence of moveable cranial bones. From his studies, Sutherland founded cranial osteopathy.

Following Sutherland's work, osteopathic physician John E. Upledger developed CranioSacral Therapy. This approach aims to release tension not only at the various points where the craniosacral bones meet, but also on the *meninges,* which are the membranes of the cerebrospinal area. His scientific studies, conducted at Michigan State University from 1975 to 1983, validated the existence of the human body's craniosacral system and its capacity to help evaluate and treat dysfunction and pain.

## *Osteopathy*

*Osteopathy* is a branch of medicine founded in 1874 by Andrew Taylor Still, an American physician who initially trained as an engineer and then attended medical college at the Kansas City School of Physicians and Surgeons. He developed a philosophy of medicine that promotes the body's natural healing powers. A doctor of osteopathy (D.O.) primarily uses manipulation therapy to restore proper body structure, allowing optimal mobility and flexibility, relieving pain, and improving overall health.

## CONDITIONS THAT RESPOND BEST

CranioSacral Therapy can be helpful in relieving or reducing the following conditions:

- Anxiety
- Attention deficit disorder (ADD)
- Central nervous system disorders
- Chronic ear infections
- Chronic fatigue

- Deafness
- Depression
- Eye problems
- Facial pain
- Headaches
- Hyperactivity

- Motor coordination difficulties
- Neck and back pain
- Sinusitis
- Temporomandibular joint (TMJ) dysfunction

## HOW DOES IT WORK?

Each person has a palpable craniosacral rhythm, and a trained practitioner can feel this subtle movement when his or her hands are placed on the cranium. The rhythm results from the expansion and contraction caused by the increase and decrease of cerebrospinal fluid, which is produced and reabsorbed at a regular rate. It is similar to the rhythms produced by the heart and by the rate of respiration. A CranioSacral Therapist can determine any imbalances or discrepancies in the craniosacral rhythm. An inconsistency suggests that normal body functions may be impaired. The practitioner usually helps to re-establish balanced rhythm and normal function by applying gentle pressure to the cranium with his or her hands. This pressure creates subtle manipulations that allow the release of tension at the cranial sutures (the places where the cranial bones meet) and on the meninges.

## WHAT TO EXPECT

You should expect a comfortable, professional office where privacy and confidentiality are maintained. The practitioner will take a full medical history, including examination through observation and questioning. He or she will address all relevant information, characteristics, and symptoms. CranioSacral Therapy usually takes place on a padded treatment table, in a quiet, sedate setting. You should wear loose-fitting, comfortable clothes.

This approach uses no needles, mechanical devices, or oils. Treatments are painless; the practitioner will use only gentle touch. During the session, you may reach a state of deep relaxation and peace. You may also experience a feeling of release, as tension is reduced. However, it is not uncommon for symptoms to worsen for a brief period (usually for twenty-four to forty-eight hours) following treatment. This response is the body's way of adapting to the changes that have occurred.

## COST/DURATION

*$50–$250 per session/60 minutes*

For the treatment of acute conditions, one to three sessions over a period of one to three weeks may be sufficient. More chronic conditions most likely will require weekly treatments for several months.

## CREDENTIALS/EDUCATION

*C.S.T.: CranioSacral Therapist*
*IAHP: International Association of Healthcare Professionals*

For recognition as a CranioSacral Therapist, the practitioner must successfully complete Upledger CranioSacral Therapy I and II, as well as several exams on technique, including an essay, an objective exam, and a practical/oral exam.

## HOW TO FIND A PRACTITIONER

The best way to find a CranioSacral Therapist is to contact the professional organization listed below, which will refer you to practitioners in your area. Another method is to look in the yellow pages under "CranioSacral Therapy"; "health services"; "holistic/wholistic centers"; and/or "holistic/wholistic practitioners." Also, many health professionals, such as osteopathic physicians, nurses, physical therapists, occupational therapists, chiropractors, and massage therapists, incorporate CranioSacral Therapy into their practices.

## PROFESSIONAL ORGANIZATION

International Association of Healthcare Practitioners (IAHP)
11211 Prosperity Farms Road, Suite D-325
Palm Beach Gardens, FL 33410-3487
(800) 311-9204 or (561) 622-4334
fax: (561) 622-4771
email: iahp@iahp.com
website: www.iahp.com

## RECOMMENDED READING

Cohen, Dan. *An Introduction to CranioSacral Therapy: Anatomy, Function and Treatment.* Berkeley, CA: North Atlantic Books, 1995.

Upledger, John B., D.O., EA.A.O. *Your Inner Physician and You: CranioSacral Therapy and Somato-Emotional Release.* Berkeley, CA: North Atlantic Books, 1997.

# EXERCISE

Exercise enables you to maintain a healthy, well-functioning body. It reduces tension and increases the sense of well-being. It enhances self-esteem, improves overall health, and makes one feel and look better. Exercise can involve cardiovascular and endurance training, stretching, and weight training. *Cardiovascular and endurance training* helps reduce body fat; decrease stress and tension; improve the functions of the lungs, heart, and blood vessels; and enhance the circulatory system's ability to supply oxygen to the tissues of the body. It can also strengthen bones and ligaments, improve sleeping patterns, and develop greater speed and stamina. Walking, running, skating, dancing, and aerobics are just a few of the many activities that promote cardiovascular health and endurance. *Stretching exercises* are excellent warm-up activities that will increase flexibility and range of motion to all the joints. Finally, *weight training* builds muscular strength to help the body withstand the activities of daily living and to prevent injury. It also develops muscle tone, endurance, and replaces fat with muscle.

Exercise approaches discussed in this book are: *aquatic therapy* (see page 24), *hatha yoga* (see page 62), *qigong* (see page 112), and *tai chi* (see page 144). In addition, approaches that incorporate at-home exercise techniques include: *chiropractic* (see page 42), *polarity therapy* (see page 98), and *the Trager approach* (see page 156).

---

## Personal Training

Personal training is a combination of fitness assessment, fitness instruction, nutritional counseling (see page 92), and motivational techniques that help you achieve physical conditioning goals. A personal trainer will design a unique program specifically for you. Motivation and positive reinforcement are emphasized, as well as proper body mechanics and the correct forms of breathing when exercising. Exercise sessions stress endurance, strength, and flexibility, while focusing attention on your personal goals and interests.

---

# THE FELDENKRAIS METHOD

## WHAT IS IT?

In order to lessen pain or discomfort, people often alter the way they hold and move their bodies. Unfortunately, such adjustments become habitual and lead to additional symptoms. The Feldenkrais Method teaches participants to become aware of movement patterns and to improve body motion. This approach endeavors to correct bad habits, alleviate pain, reduce stress, and enhance self-image. Clients learn to move with greater ease, spontaneity, and freedom, resulting in benefits to the mind, the emotions, and the entire body. The Feldenkrais Method does not attempt to change the structure of the body through adjustment or manipulation. Rather, it instructs individuals to relearn proper body movements.

Moshe Feldenkrais (1904-1984) was born in Poland and emigrated to Palestine at twelve years of age. In 1933, he received a doctorate in physics. (Feldenkrais is also known as the first European to earn a black belt in judo.) During his later life, an old soccer injury to his knees flared up. Rather than undergo surgery, Feldenkrais resolved to cure his own condition. He immersed himself in the literature of anatomy and physiology, biomechanics, and psychology. Integrating these studies with knowledge of body mechanics and his own internal awareness, Feldenkrais discovered a way to heal his knees simply by practicing proper movements. This process of self-rehabilitation was the initial step in the development of movement education. For thirty years, Feldenkrais continued to refine and teach his technique to thousands of students throughout the world.

## CONDITIONS THAT RESPOND BEST

The Feldenkrais Method is an appropriate treatment option for a number of conditions, including:

- Arthritis
- Backaches
- Bursitis
- Cerebral palsy
- Concentration problems
- Coordination problems
- Digestive difficulties
- Headaches
- Lack of endurance
- Multiple sclerosis
- Musculoskeletal disorders
- Polio
- Respiratory difficulties
- Stress-related disorders

## HOW DOES IT WORK?

The Feldenkrais Method can be taught in either group or individual sessions. Classes offer effective alternatives to unconscious, destructive habits of poor posture and improper motion. The group sessions, called *Awareness Through Movement*, teach gentle and relaxing movements. The instructor leads the class through a series of simple exercises that are performed while sitting or lying down. For example, the class may be asked to flex and extend the left foot and then to repeat the movement with the right foot. The instructor may also encourage you to imagine completing a movement before actually trying it, helping the body to function better with mindful preparation. As the class progresses, more complex movements will be introduced with the goal of helping you gain the confidence and ability to complete more challenging motions. The result is an overall sense of freer, more energized body movement.

The individual sessions, called *Functional Integration,* offer one-on-one, intensive learning. The practitioner uses passive movement techniques and manually guides you through body motions. It is a process of learning conveyed by touch. Functional Integration uses up to thirty basic positions, many of which involve lying on a firmly padded table. These private sessions are especially helpful if you have pain or are in the rehabilitative process.

## WHAT TO EXPECT

Regardless of whether you are attending group or private sessions, you should expect a safe, clean, professional, and comfortable environment. Awareness Through Movement classes are usually conducted on an exercise mat. You should wear comfortable, loose-fitting clothing that allows for flexibility. Although this is a group session, the movements are done individually and mostly in response to verbal instructions. Therefore, there is very little contact, if any.

At Functional Integration, you should expect ongoing physical contact with the practitioner, who will guide you manually through various body movements. Sessions usually take place on a low-lying, firmly-padded treatment table. Comfortable clothing that allows for free movement is recommended. The private instruction offers you a program that will be designed to suit your very specific needs.

The Feldenkrais Method uses no needles, mechanical devices, or oils. The sessions are gentle, relaxing, and relatively painless. After completing a group session, clients usually feel invigorated and experience more ease and confidence in their movements. The effects of the individual sessions vary, depending on the person and the severity of the condition being treated.

## COST/DURATION

*Individual: $60–$90 per session/approximately 45 minutes*
*Group: $15–$30 per session/approximately 45 minutes*

Concerning Awareness Through Movement, some instructors

offer drop-in classes, while others require attendance at a set number of sessions (possibly eight to twelve). The suggested number of Functional Integration sessions depends on you and your specific health needs. Some conditions require a number of weekly sessions over several months.

## CREDENTIALS/EDUCATION

*G.C.F.P.: Guild Certified Feldenkrais Practitioner*

Feldenkrais Guild® of North America (FGNA) practitioners may also use the following service marked terms:

*Awareness Through Movement*®

*Functional Integration*®

*Feldenkrais*®

*Feldenkrais Method*®

*Guild Certified Feldenkrais Practitioner*ᔆᴹ

*Guild Certified Feldenkrais Teacher*ᔆᴹ

A three–four year, professional training program accredited by the Feldenkrais Guild of North America must be completed for certification in this field. Practitioners are required to attend continuing education and to hold active practices. The Feldenkrais Method is an approach unto itself, but other healthcare professionals do incorporate it into their practices.

## HOW TO FIND A PRACTITIONER

The best way to find a Feldenkrais Method practitioner is to contact the professional organization listed below, which will refer you to instructors in your area. Another method is to look in the yellow pages under "Feldenkrais Method"; "health services"; "holistic/wholistic centers"; and/or "holistic/wholistic practitioners."

## PROFESSIONAL ORGANIZATION

Feldenkrais Guild® of North America (FGNA)
3611 SW Hood Avenue, Suite 100
Portland, OR 97201
(800) 775-2118 or (503) 221-6612

fax: (503) 221-6616
website: www.feldenkrais.com

## RECOMMENDED READING

Shafarman, Steve. *Awareness Heals: The Feldenkrais Method for Dynamic Health*. Reading, MA: Addison-Wesley, 1997.

# FLOWER ESSENCES

## WHAT IS IT?

Flowers have long been recognized for their soothing and invigorating qualities, from the pristine beauty of their colors to their intoxicating scents. Flower essences, which are liquid remedies prepared from the blossoms of fresh wildflowers, are used to treat emotional states and personality patterns. This approach does not target specific *physical* illnesses or symptoms. Rather, the client discusses his or her feelings and personality type so that the practitioner can recommend a flower essence with the capacity to change a distressing *emotional* condition.

Flower essences were popularized by Edward Bach, an English medical doctor and homeopathic physician, in the 1930s. Bach was committed to developing a gentle healing method that would address the individual's mental and spiritual nature. As part of his research, he gathered wildflowers from the English countryside and tested the healing effects of these plants on various emotional states. Bach identified thirty-eight wildflower remedies. Since that time, essences have been developed from flowers that are native to other countries, particularly from the North American region, but Bach's formulations are still the most recognized remedies.

## CONDITIONS THAT RESPOND BEST

Anyone experiencing emotional distress/turmoil may benefit from flower essences. Just a few of the conditions toward which this approach can be helpful are:

- Acute reactions to accidents and injuries
- Anxiety
- Bereavement

- Blocked emotional patterns
- Deep-rooted conflicts
- Stress-related disorders

Also, individuals who are interested in supplementing their health maintenance regimen in order to prevent future emotional or physical problems may want to consider this approach. Flower essences are effective for prevention and as adjuncts to other therapies. They are not appropriate or recommended for the treatment of severe mental health disorders such as psychoses.

## HOW DOES IT WORK?

The flower essence approach follows the belief that mental and emotional states strongly influence physical condition. Preparations are developed to gently resolve emotional distress. When the body is emotionally balanced, it is better able to cope with stress. And when stress is managed in a healthy manner, physical health improves and future illnesses can be prevented.

The majority of essences are prepared through a method originally developed by Bach. Flower blossoms in full bloom, covered with morning dew, are gathered and placed in spring water. After being exposed to bright sunlight for several hours, the blossoms are taken out and the solution is further diluted. No trace of the actual flower blossom remains in the solution.

Each type of flower has a particular healing or soothing effect, and each is applied toward specific emotions and personality patterns. The flower essence approach considers every flower to hold a unique vibration that is absorbed by the spring water. These subtle vibrations are the positive qualities needed by the individual to change negative emotional states. It is essential to select an appropriate remedy. Using an inappropriate essence will not harm you, but will not provide a significant healing effect either.

A flower essence remedy can be administered in a number of ways. Generally, several drops of the essence are used. They may be placed under the tongue or taken in a beverage. They may also be applied directly to the temples, behind the ears, on the wrists, elbows, or knees. The goal is to have the solution enter the body through ingestion or absorption. These solutions are extremely diluted and practically odorless. Unlike aromatherapy (see page 28), the scent of the flower is not part of the remedy. It is the flower's essence, taken into the body, that evokes the healing effect. The remedy is usually taken daily, often a number of times over the course of the day. Flower essence solutions are considered extremely gentle, nonaddicting, and without unpleasant side effects.

## WHAT TO EXPECT

At your consultation, you will be asked specific questions about your feelings and personality type. A single remedy (the use of one wildflower essence) or combined remedies (the use of a number of wildflower essences) will be chosen to affect your emotional condition, mood, and temperament. Over time, in response to the treatment, you are likely to feel more relaxed, better focused, and have more energy to cope with your daily routine. Once the desired improvement in emotional health has been accomplished, the remedy will not need to be taken.

For self-therapy, flower essences can be purchased at health food markets or alternative health product stores. Self-help guides and questionnaires are available to assist you in choosing an appropriate remedy.

## COST/DURATION

*Initial Session: $60–$75 (for consultation and dosage bottle)*
*Follow-up Session: $45–$60*

Length of sessions vary, depending on the emotional condition being targeted. Although some psychological conditions require longer treatment, one to twelve weeks of flower essence therapy can generally be expected to clear the emotional distress.

Fees for purchasing flower essences for self-therapy vary from store to store and depend on the specific essence.

## CREDENTIALS/EDUCATION

There are currently no licensing procedures or accrediting boards for the practice of flower essence therapy in the United States, nor any schools that have their own certification standards. Training is conducted by the Flower Essence Society and Nelson Bach USA. Many holistic professionals incorporate flower essence therapy into their practices. It is recommended that you seek a practitioner who is appropriately licensed in his or her discipline, and who has additional training in the flower essence approach.

## HOW TO FIND A PRACTITIONER

The best way to find a flower essence therapist is to contact the organizations listed below, which will refer you to practitioners in your area. Another method is to look in the yellow pages under "flower essence"; "health services"; "holistic/wholistic centers"; and/or "holistic/wholistic practitioners."

## PROFESSIONAL ORGANIZATIONS

Flower Essence Society (FES)
P.O. Box 459
Nevada City, CA 95959
(800) 736-9222 or (530) 265-9163
fax: (530) 265-0584
email: mail@flowersociety.org
website: www.flowersociety.org

Nelson Bach USA
Educational Programs
100 Research Drive
Wilmington, MA 01887
(800) 334-0843 or (978) 988-3833
fax: (978) 988-0233
email: education@nelsonbach.com
website: www.nelsonbach.com

## RECOMMENDED READING

Williamson, Vivien. *Bach Remedies and Other Flower Essences.* New York, NY: Lorenz Books, Anness Publishing, Inc., 2000.

# FOOT REFLEXOLOGY

## WHAT IS IT?

Foot reflexology is an approach that applies pressure to specific reflex areas on the feet in order to locate and correct problems in the body. It is a healing method that dates back to the ancient cultures of China, Japan, Egypt, North and South America, and India. In the early 1900s, Dr. William Fitzgerald developed a particular type of reflexology called *zone therapy.* According to Dr. Fitzgerald, the body is divided into ten equal zones. These zones extend the entire length of the body, head to toe. It follows, therefore, that when a practitioner stimulates a specific area on the foot, other parts of the body that are included in that zone will be affected. Eunice Ingham (1889-1974), a physical therapist, developed foot reflexology from the philosophy of zone therapy. Concentrating on the foot as the central area to be treated, she formulated charts that show how the entire body can be represented on the soles of the feet.

## CONDITIONS THAT RESPOND BEST

Foot reflexology can contribute to the maintenance of general health and improve the function of bodily systems. It can also help to relieve and/or reduce the following conditions:

- Allergies
- Asthma
- Balance, coordination disorders
- Bronchitis
- Cold sores
- Colds
- Colic
- Constipation
- Cramps
- Digestive problems
- Eczema
- Fatigue
- Headaches
- Hemorrhoids
- High blood pressure
- Indigestion
- Insomnia
- Lack of energy
- Lumbago
- Menopause
- Nausea

- Neuralgia
- Psoriasis
- Sinusitis

- Stiffness and soreness
- Stress-related disorders
- Ulcers

## HOW DOES IT WORK?

The goal of foot reflexology is to restore the natural flow of energy in the zones of the body by stimulating certain reflex points on the foot. For example, zone one includes the big toe and anything along the path from the toe as it travels up to the head and down the back. The thumb is also included in zone one, as the arms are represented in a manner similar to the legs. Any tightening or restriction in a muscle or tissue affects the free flow of energy throughout the entire zone. Treating areas of the feet can stimulate all the zones of the body and restore equilibrium throughout the system. In addition, very specific regions can be targeted. For example, if you suffer from a liver ailment, applying pressure to the point on the foot that is associated with the liver will actually aid in restoring proper function to that organ.

The practitioner uses stroking and sustained pressure. He or she firmly but gently strokes the soles of the feet, in order to relieve tension areas. Then pressure is applied, mostly with the thumb, to specific spots that *reflex* to the area where a problem originates. The degree of pressure varies according to sensitivity.

## WHAT TO EXPECT

You should expect a comfortable, clean environment that offers a peaceful setting. First, the practitioner will record your full medical history. Then, upon removal of socks and shoes, you will either sit in a reclining chair or lie down, with your legs supported, on a padded treatment table. The foot reflexologist is likely to examine the feet for any open sores or cuts that should be avoided during the treatment. He or she will also take note of any calluses, corns, swellings, deformities, tight areas, and the overall flexibility of the feet. Practitioners of this field are trained to assess health problems based on the tensions and sensitivities of the feet. Throughout treatment, there should be clear communication regarding the comfort level of applied pressure. While techniques are gentle, there may be areas of the feet that are sensitive or painful.

During the session, you might feel lightheaded, but this sensation will soon be replaced with deep relaxation. Upon completion, the practitioner may call attention to specific areas of sensitivity and make further treatment recommendations. The benefits of foot reflexology accumulate over a number of sessions, so results will be best after several weekly visits.

## COST/DURATION

*$60–$80 per session/45–60 minutes*

As mentioned above, the positive results of reflexology build over several treatments. Therefore, plan on arranging a number of sessions with your practitioner.

## CREDENTIALS/EDUCATION

*Certified in the Original Ingham Method*

A certified foot reflexologist is required to have completed a 200-hour program, which includes 100 hours of documented clinical work, and also must have successfully completed both a written and a practical exam. Foot reflexology is an independent field, but various healthcare practitioners incorporate this approach into their work.

Individuals who meet the educational requirements of the National Certification Board for Therapeutic Massage and Bodywork (NCBTMB) may also sit for their exam.

## HOW TO FIND A PRACTITIONER

The best way to find a foot reflexologist is to contact the professional organizations listed below, which will refer you to practitioners in your area. Another method is to look in the yellow pages under "reflexology"; "reflex zone therapy"; "zone therapy"; "health services"; "holistic/wholistic centers"; and/or "holistic/wholistic practitioners." Also, inquire into the training

of the massage therapists in your area, as some are likely to have
been trained in foot reflexology. (For information on massage, see
page 87.)

## PROFESSIONAL ORGANIZATIONS

International Institute of Reflexology, Inc.
5650 First Avenue, North
P.O. Box 12642
St. Petersburg, FL 33733-2642
(727) 343-4811
fax: (727) 381-2807
email: iir@tampabay.rr.com
website: www.reflexology-usa.net

National Certification Board for Therapeutic Massage
   and Bodywork
8201 Greensboro Drive, Suite 300
McLean, VA 22102
(800) 296-0664 or (703) 610-9015
fax: (703) 610-9005
email: info@ncbtmb.com
website: www.ncbtmb.com

## RECOMMENDED READING

Carter, Mildred, and Tammy Weber. *Healing Yourself with Foot
Reflexology: All Natural Relief from Dozens of Ailments.* Englewood
Cliffs, NJ: Prentice Hall, 1997.

Whichello Brown, Denise. *Reflexology Basics.* New York: Sterling
Publishing Co., Inc., 2001.

# HATHA YOGA

## WHAT IS IT?

Hatha yoga uses stretching and breathing exercises (see page 50),
body postures, and relaxation/meditation techniques (see page

119) to promote fitness. It is the most common form of yoga practiced in the Western Hemisphere today. Dating back more than 5,000 years, hatha yoga has not only survived, but has flourished in its ability to relieve chronic aches and pains in the human body. Present-day hatha yoga practice has developed into many forms. These range from power yoga, which is very strenuous and works almost every muscle in the body, to easy yoga, which involves chair exercises and is very passive. The goal of hatha yoga is to invigorate the body, clear the mind, and release the emotions. Because it is a gentle approach to healing the whole person, hatha yoga classes are appropriate for anyone, including individuals with physical limitations.

## CONDITIONS THAT RESPOND BEST

Hatha yoga is an appropriate option for the relief and/or reduction of the following conditions:

- Arthritis
- Asthma
- Back pain
- Headaches
- Insomnia
- Sciatica
- Stress-related disorders

This approach also provides many health benefits, including:

- Improvement of balance, coordination
- Improvement of circulation
- Improvement of concentration
- Improvement of flexibility
- Increase in endurance
- Increase in physical strength
- Increase in range of motion
- Stabilization of metabolism
- Strengthening of immunity
- Toning of internal organs

## HOW DOES IT WORK?

During a hatha yoga session, you are led through guided relaxation/meditation, breathing exercises, and stretching and toning exercises. The meditation techniques and breathing exercises reduce stress, increase circulation, and generally relax the system so that it functions more efficiently. The stretching postures open energy pathways, so that chronic blocks dissolve, energy circulates throughout the body once more, and flexibility and endurance improve. Hatha yoga provides a balanced, disciplined workout that releases muscle tension, tones the internal organs, and energizes the mind, body, and spirit. Thus, natural healing can take place.

Hatha yoga classes are conducted in small or large groups. A typical class begins with fifteen minutes of breathing exercises, followed by the stretching and toning techniques. As previously mentioned, this approach is taught at many levels. Introduction to Hatha Yoga is the most appropriate class for beginners, since postures and stretching will be simple and easy to achieve.

## WHAT TO EXPECT

The hatha yoga class should be held in a clean, relaxing environment. You should wear comfortable, loose-fitting clothing that allows for easy movement. It is advisable to bring a mat for floor work, if the instructor does not provide one. The ability to stretch and achieve various postures will develop gradually. Initially, you are likely to feel some soreness of muscles, but over time and with a commitment to practice, you will develop increased flexibility, strength, and endurance to hold a posture.

For the most part, classes will be titled "Yoga," not necessarily "Hatha Yoga." Most classes teach body postures, stretching, and meditation techniques that are gentle and simple enough to reach the majority of body types and conditions. However, attending an introductory class is your most effective evaluation technique. After the initial session, you can assess whether the particular program is suitable for your needs.

## COST/DURATION

*$15–$30 per class/60–90 minutes*

A hatha yoga program extends over a number of weeks, involving possibly eight to twelve sessions. As mentioned above, goals are gained gradually; there is a cumulative effect. In order to reach the maximum benefit of this approach, it is important to make a commitment to practicing the techniques.

## CREDENTIALS/EDUCATION

There is no official certification for hatha yoga instructors. They are trained by yoga masters over a number of years. It is recommended that you try one introductory class for evaluation purposes, to find out whether or not you are comfortable with the instructor and the level of the course. During the initial session, you can also inquire about the instructor's experience, and question other participants on their experience with him or her. Remember that the most important factor in selecting a hatha yoga program is finding a positive connection with the instructor. In addition, hatha yoga programs are available on videotape for at-home instruction.

## HOW TO FIND A PRACTITIONER

The best way to find a hatha yoga instructor is to contact the professional organization listed below, which will refer you to appropriate professionals in your area. Another method is to look in the yellow pages under "yoga"; "health services"; "holistic/wholistic centers"; "holistic/wholistic practitioners"; and/or "YMCA/YWCA."

## PROFESSIONAL ORGANIZATION

International Association of Yoga Therapists (IAYT)
2400A County Center Drive
Santa Rosa, CA 95403
(707) 566-9000
email: mail@iayt.org
website: www.iayt.org
(IAYT is a special division of Yoga Research and Education
   Center)

## RECOMMENDED READING

Baker, Jan. *Yoga for Real People*. York Beach, ME: Red Wheel/Weiser, LLC, 2002.

Carrico, Mara. *Yoga Basics: The Essential Beginners Guide to Yoga for a Lifetime of Health and Fitness.* New York: Henry Holt, 1997.

Kean, Frances and Voorhees, Susan. *A Simple Guide to Yoga.* White Plains, NY: Peter Pauper Press, 2002.

# HERBAL MEDICINE

## WHAT IS IT?

Throughout history, people have turned to plants not only for food, shelter, and clothing, but also when confronted with disease and pain. Herbal medicine uses the roots, stems, leaves, and flowers of plants for medicinal purposes. Over time and through trial and error, herbal medicine expanded into an effective system of health care. However, with the development of chemically manufactured substances, this approach did become somewhat obsolete. Yet today, as we look for safer healing techniques with fewer side effects, many individuals are turning back to the natural healing properties of plants.

## CONDITIONS THAT RESPOND BEST

The use of herbal medicine is appropriate for a wide range of illnesses that are frequently treated by conventional medicine. It is also effective as a preventive measure, providing vitamins and nutrients that enhance wellness and physical functioning. The following are examples of common conditions that herbal medicine can relieve and/or reduce:

- Acne
- Allergies
- Anxiety
- Arthritis
- Asthma
- Balance, coordination difficulties
- Cardiovascular disorders
- Circulatory disorders
- Digestive disorders
- Eating disorders
- Eczema
- Endocrine disorders

- Eye, ear, nose, throat problems
- Hay fever
- Headaches
- Immune disorders
- Insomnia
- Musculoskeletal disorders
- Nervous system disorders
- Premenstrual syndrome (PMS)
- Psoriasis
- Reproductive disorders
- Respiratory disorders
- Substance abuse
- Teeth, jaw conditions
- Varicose veins

## HOW DOES IT WORK?

The property and function of an herb dictate its application. The *property* refers to how it works, while the *function* describes for what it is used. For example, ginger has the property of a stimulant that activates the salivary glands. Its function is to remedy a dry, sore throat. Herbs can be chosen to prevent disease or to increase well-being. Often, an herbalist prescribes a combination remedy, rather than a single herb.

The goal of this approach is to develop or maintain good health by choosing herbs that work with the various body systems. Improper nutrition, lack of exercise, and/or stress can often lead to a stagnant build-up of toxins in the organs and muscles. The practitioner creates a plant remedy that induces a detoxification response. In addition, the herbs strengthen and build tissue by supplying nutrients that help repair and restore the body. Herbs are prescribed in various forms—pills, teas, liquid tinctures, creams, ointments—depending on the targeted condition.

## WHAT TO EXPECT

During the first visit, the herbalist will record your full medical history and address all relevant information, characteristics, and symptoms. Depending on his or her background and type of medical practice—for example, Ayurveda (see page 33), naturopathy (see page 88), or Traditional Chinese Medicine (see page 151)—the practitioner may use additional forms of analysis, such as blood pressure monitoring, pulse diagnosis, or iridology (eye diagnosis). The herbalist might also discuss diet and lifestyle. Then, a remedy will be formulated.

Your physical, emotional, and psychological states determine the properties and functions of the herbs, as well as the form of the remedy. The dosage and type of herbal prescription may change as your condition responds to the healing process. While herbs are generally regarded as safe, side effects can occur and should be discussed with the herbalist at the time of treatment. The practitioner will also instruct you on proper dosage and administration. Follow-up visits, if necessary, usually take place approximately two to three weeks later.

## COST/DURATION

*Initial Session: $45–$75/30–60 minutes*

Follow-up visits are generally less expensive and last only ten to fifteen minutes. Cost varies greatly, depending on the practitioner and the selected remedy. Herbal treatments are often adjuncts to other therapies, in which cases there will be additional fees.

Many individuals research and organize their own herbal health care regimens. Herbal teas are a cost-effective and simple way to begin a self-care program. For example, peppermint tea, when drank after a meal, aids the digestion process. And drinking a cup of chamomile tea is a wonderful nighttime ritual that will help the body and the mind to relax.

## CREDENTIALS/EDUCATION

*Diplomate in Chinese Herbology (NCCAOM)*
*Dipl. C.H. (NCCAOM)*

There are currently no licensing procedures or accrediting boards for the practice of herbal medicine in the United States. Various holistic/wholistic professionals—particularly Ayurvedic therapists, naturopaths, and practitioners of Traditional Chinese Medicine—use herbal remedies as part of their healing treatments. Refer to the specific sections on these approaches for information on cost/duration of treatment and applicable credentials. (Page numbers are provided earlier in this section.)

The National Certification Commission for Acupuncture and

Oriental Medicine (NCCAOM) does offer certification in Chinese Herbology. Practitioners are required to complete a minimum of 2,175 hours of training and pass the Chinese Herbology exam provided by NCCAOM. Practitioners may then designate themselves as "Diplomate in Chinese Herbology (NCCAOM)" or "Dipl. C.H. (NCCAOM)."

## HOW TO FIND A PRACTITIONER

The best way to find an herbalist is to contact the professional organizations listed below, or those listed within the sections on Naturopathy, and Traditional Chinese Medicine. These organizations will refer you to practitioners in your area. Another method is to look in the yellow pages under "herbs, herbalists, herbal medicine"; "acupuncture"; "Ayurveda"; "Chinese medicine/Traditional Chinese Medicine"; "holistic/wholistic centers"; "holistic/wholistic practitioners"; "naturopathy"; and/or "Oriental medicine doctor."

## PROFESSIONAL ORGANIZATIONS

American Holistic Medical Association (AHMA)
12101 Menaul Blvd. N.E., Suite C
Albuquerque, NM 87112
(505) 292-7788
fax: (505) 293-7582
email: info@holisticmedicine.org
website: www.holisticmedicine.org

Acupuncture and Oriental Medicine Alliance
6405 43rd Avenue Ct. NW, Suite B
Gig Harbor, WA 98335
(253) 851-6896
fax: (253) 851-6883
website: www.aomalliance.org

National Certification Commission for Acupuncture and
    Oriental Medicine (NCCAOM)
11 Canal Center Plaza, Suite 300
Alexandria, VA 22314

(703) 548-9004
fax: (703) 548-9079
email: info@nccaom.org
website: www.nccaom.org

## RECOMMENDED READING

Blumenthal, Mark, Sr. Editor. *Herbal Medicine.* Newton, MA: Integrative Medicine Communications, 2000.

Castleman, Michael. *The New Healing Herbs.* Emmaus, PA: Rodale, Inc., 2001.

Ody, Penelope. *The Holistic Herbal Directory.* Edison, NJ: Chartwell Books, Inc., 2001.

# HOLISTIC DENTISTRY

## WHAT IS IT?

Holistic dentistry is a branch of dental medicine that employs natural oils and herbal remedies to fight infection and strengthen the body's immune response. It is practiced by licensed dentists who integrate holistic approaches into their professional dental care practices. These practitioners recognize the dangers of mercury amalgam fillings, as well as other metals used in conventional dental procedures, and will remove these toxic materials upon the patient's request. They believe that oral x-rays are often unreliable in determining specific areas of infection and that the toxins released from these infections can cause problems throughout the body. Many holistic dentists use such methods as acupuncture (see page 16), alternative gum treatment (AIPT), cold laser therapy, homeopathic remedies (see page 73), hypnosis (see page 78), and nutritional supplements (see nutritional counseling, page 92).

## CONDITIONS THAT RESPOND BEST

Holistic dentistry is an appropriate option for the following:

- Dental phobias
- General dental maintenance
- Nontoxic cavity care
- Oral bacteria and infection
- Oral inflammation and wounds

For dental phobia treatment, you may wish to seek a holistic dentist who is certified in hypnotherapy, since that approach can help to alleviate the anxiety and stress of dental visits.

## HOW DOES IT WORK?

The holistic dentist will select a procedure according to your specific dental problem and its extent. Several treatment options are described below.

*Acupuncture* can be used to treat pain, as well as to diagnose infected areas. Fine needles are inserted at specific points on the body, stimulating a response.

*Anti-Infective Periodontal Therapy (AIPT)*, or *alternative gum treatment,* aims to remove plaque at its source. During the measurement of tooth-pocket depth and the exam of soft tissue, plaque samples from the deepest point of the pocket are removed for microscopic evaluation and then analyzed. The conservative removal of disease-causing bacteria is the goal of AIPT.

*Homeopathy* prescribes natural medications that alleviate dental pain; reduce dental disease; have antiseptic and fungicidal effects; relieve fear, anxiety, and touch sensitivity; and aid in alleviating drowsiness, upset stomach, and diarrhea. These remedies generally accelerate the symptoms and, thus, encourage the body to rid itself of the illness.

*Hypnotherapy* helps to reduce the anxiety and stress of dental phobias/dental visits. Patients become relaxed, capable of intense concentration, and open to suggestions for change.

*Cold laser therapy* kills bacteria, aids in wound healing, and decreases inflammation. This treatment is relatively painless.

*Nutritional supplements* strengthen the immune system. They work with the body's natural chemistry and generally have no side effects.

Holistic dentists endeavor to use the most natural substances and treatments possible, while providing comfort and maximizing healing potential. They take into consideration your overall state of health.

## WHAT TO EXPECT

You should expect a safe and clean environment where the latest safety precautions and tools are used. The dentist will ask you to fill out a medical history and will inquire about your experiences with bleeding, pain tolerance, and phobias or fears regarding dental work. It is recommended that you first have a consultation with the dentist. During the initial session, he or she can fully explain the appropriate procedures and options, and you can learn whether or not the doctor possesses the necessary specialty skills. A given holistic dentist will not practice *all* of the holistic procedures. A practitioner is likely to develop a specialty in one or more types of treatment.

Cleaning procedures used in holistic dentistry are very similar to those performed during a traditional dental visit, but cleaning substances are generally all-natural. Keep in mind that bacteria or infection in the oral cavity can cause symptoms in other parts of the body, including earaches, headaches, sore throats, nausea, and emotional distress. Inform the dentist if you are experiencing any of these conditions.

## COST/DURATION

*$75–$120 per visit*

The above is an approximate range of cost for a visit to a holistic dentist. However, rates and duration of holistic dental treatment vary greatly, depending on the dentist and the condition. Call the individual practitioner for specific information. A general maintenance visit with a holistic dentist will cost approximately the same amount as a regular check-up and cleaning with a conventional dentist.

## CREDENTIALS/EDUCATION

*D.D.S.: Doctor of Dental Surgery*
*D.M.D.: Doctor of Medical Dentistry*

Holistic dentists have had the same medical training and have accomplished the same degree requirements as conventional dentists. They simply have decided to employ holistic approaches and further specialize themselves in specific treatments. Their credentials should always be met with additional training in the specific alternative medicine approach utilized. Refer to the discussions on acupuncture, hypnotherapy, and nutritional counseling for further information on professional training. (Page numbers are given at the beginning of this approach section.)

## HOW TO FIND A PRACTITIONER

The best way to locate a holistic dentist is to contact the professional organization listed below, which will refer you to practitioners in your area. You could also visit the website www.dentalfind.com and select holistic dentistry. Another method is to look in the yellow pages under "holistic dentists" or "dentists."

## PROFESSIONAL ORGANIZATION

Foundation for Toxic Free Dentistry (FTFD)
P.O. Box 608010
Orlando, FL 32860-8010
(send a 78-cent #10 SASE for information on holistic dentists)

## RECOMMENDED READING

Parsa-Stay, Flora, D.D.S. *The Complete Book of Dental Remedies: A Guide to Safe and Effective Relief from the Most Common Dental Problems Using Homeopathy, Nutritional Supplements, Herbs, and Conventional Dental Care.* Garden City Park, NY: Avery Publishing Group, 1996.

# HOMEOPATHY

## WHAT IS IT?

Often, the conventional "treatment" of symptoms actually involves a suppressing of them. The body's need to eliminate these symptoms will lead to unwanted side effects and cause the condition to go deeper into the body. As a result, the illness becomes more difficult to cure. Homeopathy understands symptoms as the body's attempt to heal itself; symptoms are considered signals that indicate the body is working to restore natural balance. Therefore, homeopathic remedies, prepared from plant, animal, and mineral substances, encourage symptoms to run their course instead of suppressing them. This process stimulates the immune system, accelerates healing, and ultimately strengthens the body.

The term *homeopathy* originates from the Greek words *homeo* and *pathos,* meaning "similar" and "suffering/disease" respectively. Dr. Samuel Hahnemann (1755-1843), a German physician, is considered the father of today's homeopathic philosophy. Due to his outrage and protest against the practice of bloodletting, Hahnemann was ostracized from the medical profession and eventually left it. Working as a translator of medical books, he became familiar with the ancient *Law of Similars.* This law states that a substance taken in large amounts by a healthy person would cause illness or a set of uncomfortable symptoms, but if taken in minuscule amounts by a sick person, the same substance would benefit the body through the acceleration of healing. Hahnemann believed that effective medicine should trigger symptoms that are similar to the illness itself, thus activating and strengthening the body's immune system. He trusted in the body's natural healing abilities and felt medications that suppress or disguise symptoms should be avoided.

## CONDITIONS THAT RESPOND BEST

Homeopathic treatments are appropriate for a wide range of conditions, including:

- Acute infection
- Ailments of infants and children
- Ailments of pregnant and lactating women
- Allergies
- Anxiety
- Arthritis
- Asthma
- Back pain after childbirth

- Balance, coordination disorders
- Cardiovascular disorders
- Circulatory disorders
- Digestive disorders
- Endocrine disorders
- Headaches
- Infectious diseases
- Pain
- Relief of muscular aches and pains
- Sinusitis
- Skin eruptions
- Substance abuse

## HOW DOES IT WORK?

The best way to describe how homeopathy works is to provide an example. An individual with a cold may have a terrible, persistent cough. Each time that person coughs, he or she brings up phlegm. The body is actually defending itself, trying to rid the respiratory system of the unwanted mucous. However, the cough is disruptive, and so the person tries to eliminate it by taking a cough suppressant. The medication does not help in overcoming the virus; it only blocks the symptoms. Quite differently, a homeopathic remedy would bolster the body's natural healing system by encouraging symptoms to run their course in an accelerated manner. A medicine containing an extremely small amount of a substance that naturally produces symptoms similar to the cold virus would be administered. The body would then be prompted to remove the virus from the system. Thus, homeopathy helps the body fight the virus more effectively, rather than mask the symptoms.

Homeopathic remedies assign only extremely small doses. The original base substance must go through a series of *dilutions* in alcohol or water. Between every stage of dilution, the remedy is shaken to agitate the molecules and, therefore, activate the medication. This process is called *potentization*. Without the shaking procedure, the medicine would be ineffective. According to the *Law of Potentization*, the more a medicine is diluted and shaken, the greater its potency and effect when combating an illness.

The stronger homeopathic remedies are prescribed by trained practitioners, while the milder ones can be purchased at retail stores. But, at any level of dilution, the medicine contained in the treatment is in such a minute quantity that homeopathic remedies are considered nontoxic and free of side effects.

Today, the most common form of homeopathic medicines are tiny pills that dissolve when placed under the tongue. They are made from all-natural substances, including plants, roots, and minerals. These substances act like jumper cables, stimulating the body's healing response. The various strength levels of homeopathic remedies are indicated on the packaging. In general, the higher numbers indicate more levels of dilution and, hence, a stronger remedy. The necessary strength and dosage amount is specific to each person being treated.

---

## How to Take Homeopathic Remedies

Homeopathic remedies are formulated as small, round pellets which are contained in a pellet dispenser or as tablets. Pellets should be taken between meals, at least fifteen minutes before, or fifteen minutes after eating.

The mouth should be clean and free of any substance that may interfere with the remedy and prevent it from working—especially coffee, all camphor products, mint, menthol, eucalyptus, and all over-the-counter pharmaceuticals.

Avoid handling the tablets or pellets. They should be tapped out of the container into the cap, clean spoon, or a small piece of clean paper—then poured directly into the mouth. Contact with skin may interfere with the potency of the remedy. Discard any remedies that spill.

Remedies should be allowed to dissolve in the mouth. Patients should avoid swallowing, and when drops are administered, they should be placed directly under the tongue or mixed in a glass of water.

All homeopathic remedies should be kept away from heat above 115°F. Keep bottles tightly capped and stored at room temperature or in a dry place out of direct sunlight.

---

## WHAT TO EXPECT

You should expect a comfortable, professional office where privacy and confidentiality are maintained. The practitioner will take a full medical history, including examination through observation and questioning. All relevant information, characteristics, and symptoms will be addressed. The practitioner will also make an assessment of your vitality—your underlying strength and energy. This is especially important in prescribing the dosage of the remedy. Too low of a dosage will have little effect, and too high of a dosage could aggravate symptoms. A homeopathic remedy will be prescribed based on the outcome of this session. Follow-up visits will be scheduled in order to evaluate your response to the prescribed treatment.

It is important to be aware that some worsening of symptoms may occur in an initial reaction to the homeopathic remedy, but this response should be minimal. In most instances, there will be no noticeable aggravation if the correct dosage is taken.

## COST/DURATION

*Initial Visit: $100–$140/60 minutes*
*Follow-up Visit: $60 (average fee)/20–30 minutes*

The necessary number of sessions with your practitioner will depend upon your specific illness and cannot be anticipated here. The cost of the remedy may not be included in the general fee.

## CREDENTIALS/EDUCATION

*C.C.H.: Certified in Classical Homeopathy*
*D.Ht.: Diplomate in Homeotherapeutics*
*D.H.A.N.P.: Diplomate in Homeopathic Academy of Naturopathic*
*Physicians*

The D.Ht. credential is given only to medical doctors (M.D.s) and doctors of osteopathy (D.O.s). These practitioners must pass a written and practical competency exam. The D.H.A.N.P. is given to Naturopathic Physicians. Both of these have board certifications.

In order to be certified and receive the C.C.H. credential, candidates must have 500 hours of training and one to two years of experience before they are permitted to take a qualifying exam, which involves assessment through written and practical testing.

## HOW TO FIND A PRACTITIONER

One way to find a practitioner of homeopathy is to contact the professional organization listed below, which will supply you with information and the names of homeopathic practitioners in your area. Another method is to look in the yellow pages under "homeopathy"; "health services"; "holistic/wholistic centers"; and/or "holistic/wholistic practitioners."

## PROFESSIONAL ORGANIZATION

National Center for Homeopathy
801 N. Fairfax Street, Suite 306
Alexandria, VA 22314
(877) 624-0613 or (703) 548-7790
fax: (703) 548-7792
email: info@homeopathic.org
website: www.homeopathic.org

## RECOMMENDED READING

Lockie, Andrew, Dr. *Natural Health Encyclopedia of Homeopathy.* New York: Dorling Kindersley, 2000.

Ullman, Dana. *Homeopathy A-Z.* Carlsbad, CA: Hay House, Inc., 1999.

# HYPNOTHERAPY

## WHAT IS IT?

Hypnotherapy is an approach during which the therapist guides the client into a trance-like state called *hypnosis*. This state can be induced through several simple techniques, among which are verbal suggestions, and having the patient observe a continuously moving object. In the hypnotic state, the client becomes relaxed, capable of intense concentration, and open to suggestions for change.

The practice of hypnotherapy dates back to the ancient civilizations of China and Egypt, where it was included as part of surgical procedure. Since then, many practitioners have used and further developed hypnotherapy techniques. Franz Anton Mesmer (1734–1815), an Austrian physician who is considered the father of modern hypnotherapy, believed that stars, animals, and iron had magnetic qualities that could have strong effects on mental states. He developed treatment techniques based on these beliefs and, through suggestion of voice and the use of focal objects, successfully hypnotized many patients. The terms *mesmerized* and *animal magnetism* stem from his work.

James Braid (1795-1860), a surgeon from Scotland, observed Mesmer and developed his own theory and practice. In the 1840s, Braid labeled his technique *hypnotism*. He used hypnotism during surgical procedures and observed a decrease in bleeding, relief from surgical pain, a lowered mortality rate, and acceleration of the healing processes. Over the next one hundred years, hypnotherapy received considerable scientific attention and clinical application, resulting in the American Medical Association's acceptance of this therapy as a viable medical approach in 1958. Today, it is recognized as an effective technique for medical, psychological, and dental treatments.

## CONDITIONS THAT RESPOND BEST

Hypnotherapy is an appropriate treatment option for a number of conditions, including:

- Addictions (including smoking)
- Allergies
- Anxiety
- Arthritis
- Asthma
- Back pain
- Behavioral problems
- Childbirth, labor pain
- Dental problems, salivation and bleeding
- Endocrine disorders
- Fears
- Hypertension
- Insomnia
- Irritable bowel syndrome
- Migraines
- Nervous tension
- Phobias (including dental)
- Stress-related disorders
- Ulcers
- Weight problems

## HOW DOES IT WORK?

Hypnosis is a state between sleep and waking, referred to as the *alpha level,* in which you are relaxed and capable of intense concentration. Think about slowly awakening in the morning. You are still sleepy and your eyes remain closed, but you are aware of outside sounds or the ring of the alarm clock; you are not fully alert, but you have a semi-conscious connection to your surroundings. This experience is similar to the alpha level or the trance-like state induced by hypnotic technique. When in the state of hypnosis, you are very receptive to suggestions from the therapist. This will allow the practitioner to guide you toward changing habits, beliefs, or behaviors.

It is important to emphasize that although all individuals are capable of achieving an alpha state through hypnosis, there are wide differences in the degree of willingness to respond to treatment. No one can be forced into a hypnotic state against his or her will. You will be fully aware of everything that is happening, can speak as you desire, and are able to stop the trance if you feel uncomfortable. The motivation to participate in treatment and the hope that treatment will be effective are essential factors in benefiting from hypnosis. Individuals actively under the influence of drugs and/or alcohol and those with serious mental health conditions such as psychosis are usually unable to be brought into an hypnotic trance. Regardless, hypnosis is not recommended for people in such situations.

Hypnosis can be used to help you connect with earlier life events that you may have pushed from memory due to trauma or anxiety. This approach works under the assumption that physical, mental, and emotional problems stem from previous experiences. Under the relaxed state of hypnosis, you are likely to be more open to remembering past events. The psychotherapist can help you to process these memories and work toward resolution, so that present behavior will no longer be negatively affected.

Hypnotherapy is a powerful therapeutic tool that can remove resistance to an open and honest exploration of the unconscious. The left hemisphere of the brain governs the conscious mind, particularly language and logic. The right hemisphere, encompassing the unconscious mind, is associated with emotions and synthesis—the ability to pull it all together. Hypnotherapy allows communication between both sides.

## WHAT TO EXPECT

You should expect a comfortable, professional office where privacy and confidentiality are maintained. The atmosphere should be calming and the room may have subdued lighting. You will be asked to situate yourself in a sitting or reclining position. To facilitate hypnosis, the practitioner will integrate relaxation techniques (see page 119); the therapist will begin the process by creating a relaxing scene or visualization, using terms suggesting that you are drifting or floating away. Your eyes and limbs may feel heavy as you enter the trance-like state. Although you will remain fully aware of what is going on, you will feel detached. Hypnosis is similar to having a daydream— you doze off for a moment and focus on a specific topic, then instantly flash back to the ongoing activity. Remember, if you so desire, you can speak during, and may even terminate, the hypnotic state. While you are under hypnosis, the practitioner will begin offering advice for change. When finished, he or she will bring you out of the hypnotic state usually with a simple suggestion or word. You will remember what you said and what the therapist said to you.

Hypnotherapy cannot force you into doing anything that goes against your will. Prior to treatment, a reputable hypnotherapist will answer your questions concerning the procedure, introduce the specific techniques to be used, and explain that you have the control to stop the process at any time.

There is controversy over whether memories recalled under hypnosis are true memories. They may be combined with experience and feelings that were developed consciously or unconsciously over the years and, hence, cannot be guaranteed as completely accurate. The benefit of hypnosis will be in its ability to help you ultimately function more positively, effectively, and with less fear, pain, and/or hindrance from negative behaviors. You can also learn to use self-hypnosis, which combines self-relaxation techniques and the principles of hypnotic suggestion to change your behavior and attitude. Consult your practitioner regarding this possibility.

## COST/DURATION

*$60–$150 per session/30–50 minutes*

One session of hypnotherapy can be effective in helping certain conditions, but the duration and frequency of treatment will depend on your condition and your goals. The fee range given above is based on the wide variety of professionals who may use hypnotherapy.

## CREDENTIALS/EDUCATION

*C.H.: Certified Hypnotherapist*

Practitioners with the C.H. credential have completed a hypnotherapy training program approved by the American Board of Hypnotherapy, or have passed an examination approved by the same board, or have maintained a private or group practice in hypnotherapy for three years. It is recommended that you select a practitioner who has a professional license in the healing arts, such as a psychiatrist, psychologist, social worker, nurse, pastoral counselor, physician, or dentist, and who holds additional approval as a certified hypnotherapist.

The American Society of Clinical Hypnosis also offers certification in hypnosis as certification in clinical hypnosis or as an approved consultant in clinical hypnosis.

## HOW TO FIND A PRACTITIONER

The best way to find a hypnotherapist is to contact the professional organizations listed below, which will refer you to certified practitioners in your area. Another method is to look in the yellow pages under the following categories: "hypnosis"; "hypnotherapy"; "health services"; "holistic/wholistic centers"; and/or "holistic/wholistic practitioners."

## PROFESSIONAL ORGANIZATIONS

American Board of Hypnotherapy
2002 E. McFadden Avenue, Suite 100
Santa Ana, CA 92705
(800) 872-9996 or (714) 245-9340
fax: (714) 245-9881
email: info@hypnosis.com
website: www.hypnosis.com

The American Society of Clinical Hypnosis
140 N. Bloomingdale Road
Bloomingdale, IL 60108-1017
(630) 980-4740
fax: (630) 351-8490
email: info@asch.net
website: www.asch.net

International Medical and Dental Hypnotherapy Association
4110 Edgeland, Suite 800
Royal Oak, MI 48073-2285
(248) 549-5594 or (800) 257-5467
website: www.infinityinst.com

National Guild of Hypnotists
P.O. Box 308
Merrimack, NH 03054-0308
(603) 429-9438
fax: (603) 424-8066
email: ngh@ngh.net
website: www.ngh.net

## RECOMMENDED READING

Fisher, Stanley, Ph.D. *Discovering the Power of Self-Hypnosis: The Simple Natural Mind-Body Approach to Change and Healing.* New York: Newmarket Press, 2000.

Krasner, A.M., Ph.D. *The Wizard Within: The Krasner Method of Clinical Hypnotherapy.* Santa Ana, CA: American Board of Hypnotherapy Press, 1990.

# LYMPHATIC MASSAGE

## WHAT IS IT?

Touch is instinctual when it comes to providing comfort and demonstrating care. Therefore, massage—the practice of kneading or otherwise manipulating a person's muscles and other soft tissue with the intent of improving that individual's well-being—is a natural way to relax and relieve tired, sore muscles. The ancient Chinese, Greek, and Roman cultures practiced massage as part of their healing arts. Today, its therapeutic benefits continue to help many people. Lymphatic massage is one of the numerous techniques available. (For references to other types of massage, see page 87.)

In the 1930s, Dr. Emil Vodder of Denmark developed a massage technique that focused on the lymphatic system. The healthy flow of lymphatic fluid is essential, for it provides nourishment and building materials to body tissues and plays a vital role in proper immune functioning. The lymphatic system, which ultimately works to eliminate waste products from the tissues, is entirely dependent upon the external pressure from muscle contraction and joint movement that occurs during such activities as walking, running, and exercising. When the lymphatic system is sluggish due to illness, a sedentary lifestyle, or physical limitations, waste accumulates, affecting metabolism and causing fatigue. The purpose of lymphatic massage is to stimulate the lymphatic system to carry away excessive waste in the loose connective tissue by manually producing the necessary pressure. The approach is used primarily to treat specific conditions, not for general relaxation.

## CONDITIONS THAT RESPOND BEST

Lymphatic massage is a helpful approach for the relief and/or reduction of the following conditions:

- Acute edema
- Allergies
- Asthma
- Bruising

- Immune system disorders
- Minor skin ailments
- Minor sports injuries
- Muscle strains

- Chronic edema
- Fibrosis
- Headaches
- Neuromuscular disorders
- Post-mastectomy pain
- Sinus congestion

This approach is also helpful to those in the following life situations:

- Physical limitations
- Sedentary lifestyle

## HOW DOES IT WORK?

During a lymphatic massage, the practitioner applies extremely light, repetitive strokes to a specific area of the body until a very thin film of lymphatic fluid appears on the skin. This indicates that lymphatic fluid is flowing more efficiently. He or she then moves to another area of the body and repeats the process. When the massage therapist reaches a joint such as a knee or elbow, he or she steadily pumps the limb, in order to release the fluid that settles in these areas so that it can resume proper flow. The entire massage is done according to a very specific pattern, in order to direct the lymphatic fluid to the lymph nodes, where the fluid can be filtered and waste can be eliminated. The result is a decrease in muscle stiffness and soreness.

## WHAT TO EXPECT

You should expect a safe, clean environment. During your first visit, the therapist will inquire about your full medical history, so that any necessary precautions can be taken. Next, you will be asked to lie on a well-padded treatment table. It is recommended that you wear gym shorts and a T-shirt. The therapist should be especially sensitive to draping procedures, exposing only the area of the body that requires therapeutic attention. It is very important to have clear communication between you and your practitioner regarding the level of pressure applied, sensitive areas, and comfort. After treatment, you may feel somewhat lethargic and relaxed. Drinking plenty of water will help to flush the loosened toxins from your system.

If you suffer from the following conditions or situations, massage may not be an appropriate treatment, and caution is recommended: acute infectious diseases; aneurysm; cancer; fever; hematoma; hernia; high blood pressure; inflammation due to tissue damage or from bacteria; osteoporosis; phlebitis; varicose veins; or if you are intoxicated or on medication that contraindicates massage.

## COST/DURATION

*$45–$90 per session/30–60 minutes*

Acute problems can respond to a single session of lymphatic massage, whereas chronic conditions may require a regular massage schedule.

## CREDENTIALS/EDUCATION

*C.M.L.D.T.: Certified Manual Lymph Drainage Therapist*
*IAHP: International Association of Healthcare Professionals*

In order to use the credential C.M.L.D.T., a therapist should be instructed and certified by the Dr. Vodder School for Manual Lymph Drainage. As a prerequisite to this program, the student must be a trained member of an allied health profession such as massage therapy, physical therapy, or nursing. (For information on credentials regarding the general practice of massage, please refer to the *Practitioners' Credentials* section of this book, page 171.) When a practitioner uses the credential IAHP, it means they have met the educational requirements in order to join this organization.

## HOW TO FIND A PRACTITIONER

The best way to find a practitioner of lymphatic massage is to contact the professional organizations listed below, which will refer you to certified therapists in your area. It is important to note that qualified lymphatic massage practitioners are not necessarily members of these organizations. Another way to locate a lymphatic massage therapist is to look in the yellow pages under "massage"; "therapeutic massage"; "holistic/wholistic centers"; and/or "holistic/wholistic practitioners." Be sure to inquire if the practitioners specialize in lymphatic massage.

## PROFESSIONAL ORGANIZATIONS

North American Vodder Association of Lymphatic Therapy
356 Waterbury Drive
East Lake, OH 44095
(888) 462-8258
website: www.navalt.com

International Association of Healthcare Practitioners (IAHP)
11211 Prosperity Farms Road, Suite D-325
Palm Beach Gardens, FL 33410-3487
(800) 311-9204 or (561) 622-4334
fax: (561) 622-4771
email: iahp@iahp.com
website: www.iahp.com

## RECOMMENDED READING

Beck, Mark F. *Milady's Theory and Practice of Therapeutic Massage.* 2nd ed. Albany, NY: Milady Publishing Co., 1994.

# MASSAGE

Massage is the practice of kneading or manipulating a person's muscles and other soft tissue with the intent of improving that individual's well-being. Its concept is instinctual; most people immediately react to injury by rubbing the traumatized area of the body. The sensation of touch is one of the oldest and best known ways to demonstrate caring and to provide comfort. So massage is a natural way of relaxing tired, sore muscles. As a healing art, this approach dates back to the ancient Chinese, Greek, and Roman cultures. Today, massage therapy is comprised of numerous techniques. This book explores three of these: *lymphatic massage* (see page 84), *sports massage* (see page 135), and *Swedish massage* (see page 140). Please refer to the specific approach sections for further information.

If you suffer from the following conditions or situations, massage may not be an appropriate treatment, and caution is recommended: acute infectious diseases; aneurysm; bruises; cancer; fever; hematoma; hernia; high blood pressure; inflammation due to tissue damage or from bacteria; osteoporosis; phlebitis; skin conditions; varicose veins; or if you are intoxicated or on medication that contraindicates massage.

# MYOTHERAPY

Myotherapy, commonly known as trigger point therapy, is a bodywork technique that focuses on tender, congested spots on muscle tissue that radiate pain to other parts of the body. For a discussion on Trigger Point Therapy, see page 159.

# NATUROPATHY

## WHAT IS IT?

Naturopathy is best explained through its philosophies: the human body has the ability to heal itself; symptoms are not part of a disease, but are signs that the body is working to eliminate toxins; a person should be treated as a whole, taking into account physical, psychological, emotional, and genetic factors. This approach is not a single medical theory developed by any one person, but rather it is a combination of healing approaches drawn from various parts of the world. In fact, naturopathy includes wisdom from the medicines of ancient Greek, Chinese, Indian, and Native American cultures. It promotes a healthy lifestyle through exercise, relaxation, and a diet of natural, organic foods.

Naturopaths are general practitioners who specialize in natural medicine. Though most naturopaths build their practices around one or two therapeutic approaches, they are trained in many areas of medicine, including: acupuncture (see page 16); clinical nutrition (see nutritional counseling, page 92); counseling (see psychotherapy, page 103); dietary and lifestyle modifications; exercise therapy (see page 50); herbal medicine (see page 66); homeopathy (see page 73); hydrotherapy (see page 27); natural childbirth; osteopathy (see page 47); Traditional Chinese Medicine (see page 151); and, in some states, minor surgery and limited drug prescription.

## CONDITIONS THAT RESPOND BEST

Being that naturopaths are licensed primary care practitioners, any condition normally treated by a general practitioner or internist also can be managed under naturopathic care. As mentioned above, naturopaths are trained in many types of care. For a list of conditions and situations that can benefit from a specific therapy, turn to the discussion on that approach. (Page references are given at the beginning of this section.) Naturopaths generally will cooperate with and refer clients to other health professionals when it is necessary.

## HOW DOES IT WORK?

The first step in the naturopathic healing process is to determine the underlying cause of an illness. There are various reasons why a given illness might occur. For example, if you are experiencing a digestive disorder, the naturopath must determine if the illness is due to poor eating habits, to tension in the spinal area creating pressure on nerves that supply the digestive organs, or to a stressful life issue. When you experience stress, the digestive area often becomes a holding place for tension-causing emotions, resulting in digestive difficulties.

Once the cause is determined, the primary role of the naturopath is one of an educator. Teaching lifestyle changes and making recommendations on diet, exercise, and eating habits encourages self-responsibility for health. In most cases, dietary factors play a major role. Nutritional supplements and proper diet are recognized as fundamental to strengthening the internal systems of the body. Following naturopathic principles, the practitioner selects the best possible treatment plan from a wide array of healing techniques, several of which are described below.

*Acupuncture* is an ancient Chinese method of healing in which hair-thin, disposable needles are inserted into specific points on the body. The stimulation works to balance and harmonize the energy flow in the human body.

*Clinical nutrition* stresses the use of whole, natural foods and nutritional supplements for the maintenance of health and the treatment of disease. This approach to health recommends a diet of foods that are organically grown—raised without the use of chemicals and pesticides—and that have not been processed, refined, or stored for long periods of time.

*Herbal medicine* involves the use of roots, stems, flowers, and leaves of plants for medicinal purposes. Remedies can remove toxins from the body with fewer side effects than manufactured drugs, and also strengthen and build tissues by supplying nutrients.

*Homeopathy* encourages the body's natural healing response through the administration of minute doses of a remedy that produces symptoms similar to the illness itself. The treatment activates and strengthens the body's immune system.

*Hydrotherapy* involves the therapeutic use of water for healing purposes. Among the available techniques are: hot or cold baths, mineral baths, steam baths, and hot or cold body wrappings.

*Osteopathy* is a branch of medicine that uses massage and manipulation, and concentrates on the joints of the body. Special focus is given to the spinal area, as osteopaths believe that proper alignment of the vertebrae will enhance the body's natural capacity to heal itself.

*Traditional Chinese Medicine* is based on the philosophy that healing energy circulates throughout the body. The free flow of this energy is essential to good health, and can be maintained or stimulated by such treatments as acupuncture, acupressure, and herbal medicine.

Through naturopathic approaches, you play an active role in your recovery process and health maintenance. Importantly, in order for the treatments to be most effective, you must make a commitment to change. It may be necessary for you to restructure dietary and lifestyle habits in order to gain the health benefits of naturopathic care.

## WHAT TO EXPECT

You should expect a safe, clean environment where privacy and confidentiality are maintained. On your first visit, a thorough medical history will be taken, including information on your lifestyle habits, diet, occupation, and family history of disease. The practitioner might take your blood pressure and evaluate your skin, hair, nails, and eyes. In addition, the diagnosis might require lab work and/or x-rays. Treatment approaches will be discussed, as well as an at-home health maintenance program. The first visit can last as long as ninety minutes.

For the most part, your naturopath will perform the suggested treatments himself or herself, but he or she may occasionally refer to a specialist in another alternative medicine approach. Please read the sections on the specific approaches for more information on what to expect. (Page numbers are provided earlier in this section.)

## COST/DURATION

*Initial Visit: $80–$225/60–90 minutes*
*Follow-up Visit: $60–$90/30–60 minutes*

The cost and duration of treatment will vary according to the condition and to the approaches that are assigned. It is important to note that there may be additional charges for lab work and other diagnostic procedures.

## CREDENTIALS/EDUCATION

*N.D.: Doctor of Naturopathic Medicine*

Naturopaths obtain a Doctor of Naturopathic Medicine (N.D.) degree from a four-year, graduate level, naturopathic medical college. The first two years of schooling are similar to that of traditional medical school, while the last two years of training focus on naturopathic approaches with an emphasis on nutrition. Some states regulate the practice of naturopathy, in which cases candidates must also pass a state or national board examination.

## HOW TO FIND A PRACTITIONER

The best way to locate a naturopath is to contact the professional organization listed below, which will refer you to practitioners in your area. However, it is important to note that qualified naturopaths are not necessarily members of these organizations. Another way to locate a practitioner is to look in the yellow pages under "naturopathy"; "naturopathic physicians"; "health services"; and/or "holistic/wholistic practitioners."

## PROFESSIONAL ORGANIZATION

The American Association of Naturopathic Physicians
3201 New Mexico Avenue NW, Suite 350
Washington, DC 20016
(866) 538-2267 or (202) 895-1392
fax: (202) 274-1992
website: www.naturopathic.org

## RECOMMENDED READING

Weil, Andrew, M.D. *Natural Health Natural Medicine.* New York: Houghton Mifflin, 1998.

# NUTRITIONAL COUNSELING

## WHAT IS IT?

What we *should* eat and what we *do* eat are rarely the same. Many factors, from lifestyle and time constraints to culturally learned eating habits, determine our diets. Furthermore, societal pressure to look a certain way can make eating a psychological nightmare rather than an enjoyable approach to good health. But nutrition is fundamental to well-being and generally is a common denominator in every condition treated. Nutritional counseling covers a wide range of assessments and dietary philosophies. Nutritionists offer education on numerous subjects, including facts about nutrition, eating patterns, vitamins/minerals, food allergies, and weight loss. They work with clients to design individual diets that provide both variety and proper nutrition. The promotion of wellness through dietary and lifestyle recommendations can be a primary or adjunct therapy.

## CONDITIONS THAT RESPOND BEST

In addition to its role in general health maintenance, nutritional counseling is a principal part of the holistic/wholistic approach to most illnesses and medical conditions. It is especially effective for:

- Allergies
- Anemia
- Anxiety
- Arthritis
- Balance, coordination disorders
- Cancer
- Cataracts
- Chronic bloating
- Colds, general infection
- Depression
- Dermatological problems
- Diabetes
- Endocrine system disorders
- Eye, ear, nose, throat conditions
- Fatigue
- Gastrointestinal disorders
- High blood pressure
- High cholesterol levels
- Influenza
- Insomnia
- Joint, bone problems
- Low blood pressure
- Migraines or headaches
- Mood swings
- Nausea
- Obesity
- Parkinson's disease
- Pregnancy
- Premenstrual syndrome (PMS)
- Respiratory conditions
- Sinusitis
- Stress-related disorders
- Substance abuse
- Teeth, jaw conditions

## HOW DOES IT WORK?

Illnesses due to nutritional deficiencies are common. Even if you follow a diet of healthy foods, it is likely that you are not attaining maximum nutrition. One reason is that the nutritional values of foods change following cooking, processing, presenting, and storage procedures. In addition, certain prescribed medications produce vitamin deficiencies, and many over-the-counter laxatives, diuretics, and pain medications rob the body of vitamins, minerals, and vitality. Nutritional counseling designs a good nutritional regimen beginning with a planned diet that will provide the body with an adequate supply of the nutrients it needs to function properly. Whether you are trying to treat disease or you desire to increase energy and maintain good health, there are many nutritional philosophies from which to choose.

*Ayurveda* follows the philosophy that illness is a state of imbalance within the body's systems, and the goal is to obtain a healthy balance. Careful consideration will be given to your body type; each person falls under one of three body types, and treatment is arranged around this designation. Food selections also will be based on the six tastes: salty, sour, pungent, bitter, sweet, and astringent. It is recommended that all six tastes are included in each meal, even if it means a simple sprinkling of a particular spice. You will be encouraged to follow guidelines from a list of foods to eat and to avoid. (See page 33 for more information on Ayurvedic practices.)

*Clinical nutrition* stresses whole, natural foods and nutritional supplements for the maintenance of health and the treatment of disease. A diet of organically grown foods (that is, foods that have not been treated with chemicals or pesticides) that also have not been processed, refined, or stored for long periods of time is recommended. Clinical nutrition holds a place of primary importance to practitioners of naturopathic medicine. They feel that clients should be aware of the foods that can heal and provide vitality, as well as foods that can affect moods and cause stress. With proper food choices, your physical, emotional, and mental health can be maintained.

*Food allergy counseling* helps individuals to determine food hypersensitivities, allergies, or food intolerance through elimination diets. Certain foods, such as dairy, wheat, or meat, will be eliminated from your diet, in order to determine your response.

These foods are carefully reintroduced, one at a time, to determine their effects on your symptoms, behavior, and emotional state. Ultimately, the food allergist will design a diet of allergy-free foods.

*Oriental nutrition* categorizes and selects foods according to the philosophies of Traditional Chinese Medicine (TCM) and, in particular, the principle of *yin and yang*. Traditional Chinese Medicine is a holistic medicine that aims to maintain the proper flow of life energy throughout the body. (For more information on TCM, see page 151.) The principle of yin and yang states that all things are comprised of two opposite components, such as hot and cold or light and dark. One component cannot exist without the other; they are interdependent. Foods are categorized as yin or yang, and the human system needs both for healthy function. Diet also will be determined by your constitution, personality, and health, as well as the environment and climate in which you live. The overall objective of oriental nutrition is to maintain balance in the body. For example, if you always feel cold, have poor circulation, and live in a chilly environment, you will be encouraged to eat more yang food, which is warming.

*Macrobiotic counseling* extends the principles of oriental nutrition. All foods in macrobiotics are categorized as yin (cooler) or yang (warmer). The idea is to establish eating habits based on the individual's needs and environment. A low-fat, high-fiber diet consisting of whole grains, vegetables, sea vegetables, and seeds will be recommended. Foods should be seasonal and grown locally. You will be taught to slice and prepare foods in a specific manner, in order to maintain the characteristics of yin and yang, and to cook in accordance with macrobiotic principles. Participants of macrobiotics believe that illness is the result of poor nutrition, bad eating habits, and a sedentary lifestyle. Through regular exercise and eating fresh, whole foods that are synchronized with the cycles of nature, the prevention of illness and the maintenance of health can be achieved.

*Western nutrition* stresses the scientific knowledge behind the nutritional function of food, as well as the daily nutritional requirements necessary for good health. By understanding the chemical components of nutrients (proteins, sugars, fats, carbohydrates, and fiber), you will be better able to make healthy decisions about food. Nutritionists will discuss the risk factors of certain foods, including the dangers of processed, refined, and chemically treated substances. They will recommend dietary changes and instruct you on proper eating habits.

In today's fast-paced and stressful world, it is easier to eat for convenience rather than to eat for health. Having a professional nutritionist design a program specifically for you can provide much needed vitality in your life. Nutritional counseling is a natural way to take control of your life and to increase its quality.

## WHAT TO EXPECT

Your nutritional evaluation and counseling should take place in a quiet, clean environment. The nutritionist will record your medical history and ask specific questions concerning dietary intake. During the evaluation process, your nutritional needs and goals will be discussed. A program will then be designed based on your symptoms, constitution, lifestyle, and nutritional assessment. Due to the different dietary philosophies of various health practitioners, it is advisable to arrange a brief initial consultation. At this meeting, you can determine if the type of nutritional counseling that you are attending is appropriate for your needs.

## COST/DURATION

*$60–$90 per visit/30–60 minutes*

Professionals in the nutrition field generally require that their clients attend a minimum of three office visits. Additional sessions may be scheduled in order to integrate facts about nutrition into daily life routines. If supplements are recommended by the practitioner, there will be additional expenses. Vitamins, minerals, and food supplements are widely available in food markets and drug/vitamin stores. In addition, supermarkets are now offering more healthy food choices, as there is a growing demand for such products.

## CREDENTIALS/EDUCATION

*C.N.C.®: Certified Nutritional Consultant*
*(accredited by the American Association of Nutritional Consultants)*
*L.D.: Licensed Dietitian (state license)*
*N.D.: Doctor of Naturopathic Medicine*
*R.D.: Registered Dietitian*
*(accredited by the American Dietetic Association)*

Nutritional counselors can be educated in a variety of programs/ schools. In order to practice, they should have achieved one of the above titles, or be recognized practitioners of Ayurvedic (see page 33) or Traditional Chinese Medicine (see page 151).

## HOW TO FIND A PRACTITIONER

The best way to locate a nutritionist is to contact the professional organizations listed below, which will refer you to practitioners in your area. Another way to find a nutritional counselor is to look in the yellow pages under "nutritional therapy"; "nutritionist"; "Ayurveda"; "diet centers"; "dietitian"; "health clinics"; "macrobiotic counseling"; "naturopathy"; and/or "Oriental medicine." The nutrition departments of local hospitals will also provide information on practitioners.

## PROFESSIONAL ORGANIZATIONS

The American Association of Naturopathic Physicians
3201 New Mexico Avenue NW, Suite 350
Washington, DC 20016
(866) 538-2267 or (202) 895-1392
fax: (202) 274-1992
website: www.naturopathic.org

American Association of Nutritional Consultants
400 Oak Hill Drive
Winona Lake, IN 46590
(888) 828-2262
fax: (574) 269-4060
email: registrar@aanc.net
website: www.aanc.net

American Dietetic Association
120 South Riverside Plaza, Suite 2000
Chicago, IL 60606-6995
(800) 877-1600 or (312) 899-0040
website: www.eatright.org

The Ayurvedic Institute
P.O. Box 23445
Albuquerque, NM 87192-1445
(505) 291-9698
fax: (505) 294-7572
website: www.ayurveda.com

Acupuncture and Oriental Medicine Alliance (AOMA)
6405 43rd Avenue Ct. NW, Suite B
Gig Harbor, WA 98335
(253) 851-6896
fax: (253) 851-6883
website: www.aomalliance.org

## RECOMMENDED READING

Crayhon, Robert, M.S. *Nutrition Made Simple.* New York: M. Evans & Co., Inc., 1996.

# POLARITY THERAPY

## WHAT IS IT?

Energy balancing approaches restore the flow of the body's natural healing energies. Such therapies typically involve various forms of light touch to relieve pain and stress and to encourage healing. Polarity therapy is one of these approaches. It is based on the philosophy that energy flows freely in nature and that the stagnation of this energy in the human body is the underlying cause of disease. Practitioners of polarity therapy use subtle manipulations and techniques that hold, rock, or simply touch specific points. The healthy energy current that results serves to balance emotions and to promote a vital body and clear mind. The polarity therapist also instructs the client on mild exercises and stretching postures to be done at home.

Polarity therapy was developed by Randolph Stone (1890-1981), an Austrian who was a doctor of osteopathy and naturopathy, as well as a chiropractor. He found that the balancing of energy was the central concept behind many ancient and traditional healthcare systems. After sixty years of research, study, and clinical practice in acupuncture, herbology, Eastern massage, foot reflexology, shiatsu, and zone therapy, Dr. Stone assigned the term *polarity* to describe the qualities of magnetic energy that circulate throughout the body; when energy is flowing in a healthy manner, it is charged with the qualities of attraction and repulsion and, thus, is drawn toward positive and negative *poles.* During polarity therapy, the practitioner's hands provide an opposite pole, and the applied pressure stimulates energy movement. Stone also felt that wellness is achieved only through the healthy interdependence of body, mind, and spirit. Therefore, polarity therapy endeavors to improve the function of and relationship between all three.

## CONDITIONS THAT RESPOND BEST

Polarity therapy is an appropriate treatment for the following conditions:

- Abscesses
- Allergies
- Anorexia, bulimia
- Anxiety
- Arthritis
- Back and neck pain
- Balance, coordination disorders
- Boils
- Cardiovascular disorders
- Circulatory disorders
- Cold sores
- Colic
- Constipation
- Cramps
- Depression
- Eczema
- Endocrine system disorders
- Fatigue
- Fibromyalgia

- Fluid retention
- Headaches
- Hemorrhoids
- Immune system disorders
- Indigestion
- Insomnia
- Menopause

- Menstrual problems
- Nausea
- Phobias
- Psoriasis
- Respiratory problems
- Stress-related disorders
- Trauma
- Ulcers

## HOW DOES IT WORK?

In our bodies, as in all of nature, energy is characterized by the fundamental principles of attraction and repulsion. For energy to move, there must be two unobstructed, opposite fields; a positive and a negative field create a polarity relationship. When energy is blocked, it turns neutral. The surrounding body tissue stagnates, becoming either flaccid and weak or extremely tight. If the areas around the obstruction are touched, you experience a sensation of numbness or pain. Suppressed emotions, internalized stress, and poor nutrition are some of the major causes of blocked energy.

The polarity therapist generally begins with a series of finger or hand placements to help induce a state of deep relaxation and to locate stagnation. Energy blockages reside in muscles, bones, and internal organs. Then, light touch and subtle manipulations recharge the neutral areas. Pressure moves the energy and the hands of the therapist act as either positive or negative poles, creating an opposite toward which the energy is drawn. As blocked energy is released, suppressed thoughts may surface and/or a sensation of tingling, heat, or pulsation may be felt in the obstructed tissue. Yawning, coughing, profound calmness, and deep breathing are indications that an energy block has been dissolved. Restoring the healthy flow of energy "jump starts" your body and allows it to function optimally.

Polarity therapy also includes mild exercises and stretching postures called *polar energetics*. Polar energetics encourage you to participate in, and be responsible for, the maintenance of your health. These movements include squatting and scissor kicks. All exercises are based on opening energy currents in the body. They are demonstrated by the practitioner and then can be done at home.

## WHAT TO EXPECT

You should expect a safe, clean environment where privacy and confidentiality are maintained. The practitioner will record your full medical history and will address all relevant information, characteristics, and symptoms. During a polarity therapy session, you will remain fully clothed and will either sit or lie on a treatment table. It is recommended that you wear loose-fitting, cotton clothing for comfort and flexibility. Subtle manipulations and light touch will be conducted on the entire body. Generally, clients experience a deep calm during and after polarity therapy. Physical improvement is likely to occur over a number of sessions. Your commitment and motivation are key forces in your recovery.

Polarity therapists suggest that you eat only a light meal before treatment, and that you avoid stimulants such as coffee, caffeine sodas, and sugar for two hours prior to a session. During treatment, you may experience some emotional distress due to the release of repressed emotions from past trauma. If you feel overwhelmed, it may be helpful to see a licensed psychotherapist. (See page 103 for information on psychotherapy.)

## COST/DURATION

*$60–$90 per session/60 minutes*

As mentioned above, maximum benefit from polarity therapy is achieved over several sessions. Therefore, consider attending a number of treatment sessions—for example, three to twelve sessions over one to three months.

## CREDENTIALS/EDUCATION

*R.P.P.: Registered Polarity Practitioner*

In order to become a polarity therapist, practitioners must accomplish at least 615 hours of training from an American Polarity Association accredited school. This approach is an independent field, but a number of healthcare professionals from other specialties also seek training and use it as an adjunct therapy.

Individuals who meet the educational requirements of the National Certification Board for Therapeutic Massage and Bodywork (NCBTMB) may also sit for their exam.

## HOW TO FIND A PRACTITIONER

The best way to find a polarity therapist is to contact the professional organization listed below, which will refer you to a practitioner in your area or a nearby polarity training institute. Many schools offer training clinics that provide treatments at reduced rates. It is important to note that qualified polarity therapists are not necessarily members of this organization. Another way to locate a practitioner is to look in the yellow pages under "polarity therapy" or under "health services"; "holistic/wholistic centers"; and/or "holistic/wholistic practitioners."

## PROFESSIONAL ORGANIZATIONS

American Polarity Therapy Association
P.O. Box 19858
Boulder, CO 80308
(303) 545-2080
fax: (303) 545-2161
email: hq@polaritytherapy.org
website: www.polaritytherapy.org

National Certification Board for Therapeutic Massage
    and Bodywork
8201 Greensboro Drive, Suite 300
McLean, VA 22102
(800) 296-0664 or (703) 610-9015
fax: (703) 610-9005
email: info@ncbtmb.com
website: www.ncbtmb.com

## RECOMMENDED READING

Beaulieu, John, N.D., Ph.D., R.P.P. *Polarity Therapy Workbook.* New York: BioSonic Enterprises, Ltd., 1994.

# PSYCHOTHERAPY

## WHAT IS IT?

Emotions play a vital role in our lives. If they become pent-up or pushed aside, the resulting internal pressure leads to an increase in anxiety, anger, depression, dysfunctional behavior, and/or physical symptoms. Psychotherapy focuses on the healing of the mind and the emotions. It provides an attentive listener and comfortable, safe surroundings, giving the client an opportunity to identify conflicts, release emotions, and find useful coping strategies. By its very nature, psychotherapy is a holistic approach. Practitioners are trained to assess a client's functioning from physical, emotional, mental, environmental, social, and spiritual perspectives, in order to help him or her to process emotions and cope more successfully. Differences abound in the techniques used, but understanding the whole person, in terms of his or her particular strengths, limitations, and experience, is a basic tenet of every theoretical branch of psychotherapy.

For centuries, philosophers, writers, and spiritual leaders have studied the inner workings of the human mind and its emotions, as well as methods for healing its conflicts. But it was Sigmund Freud, a medical doctor and researcher from Vienna, who started the practice most closely related to present-day psychotherapy. In the late nineteenth and early twentieth centuries, Freud provided the vocabulary to describe psychological processes. He labeled the *unconscious* and developed a form of psychotherapy called *psychoanalysis,* which therapeutically explores a patient's personal history and emotions. From the establishment of this *talking cure,* other psychological theories and methods have developed. Today, there are numerous schools of psychotherapy, each with their own theoretical framework, methods, and language. Yet still, psychotherapy is a process of talking, a discussion between a trained psychotherapist and a person struggling with a life problem. The client may be seeking personal growth through a clearer understanding of the self, or may be desiring to change specific attitudes or behaviors. This approach can help him or her to build self-esteem and to improve relationships with family, friends, and/or coworkers. It can enhance his or her ability to cope with stress, loss, physical or mental illness, life-stage issues, addictions, and/or the experience of trauma.

## CONDITIONS THAT RESPOND BEST

Psychotherapy can be helpful in the treatment of many conditions, including:

- Anxiety
- Back pain
- Cardiovascular system disorders
- Chronic pain disorders
- Depression
- Eating disorders
- Impeded sports performance
- Musculoskeletal disorders
- Panic, phobias
- Stress-related disorders
- Substance abuse, addictions

This approach also promotes better health management of the following situations:

- Child, adolescent troubles
- Coping with aging parents
- Divorce
- Illness and recovery
- Life-stage issues
- Loneliness
- Low self-esteem
- Personal development, enrichment, growth
- Relationship issues
- School, work difficulties
- Trauma from death, accidents, sexual abuse, physical abuse, rape, violence

## HOW DOES IT WORK?

A psychotherapist is a trained practitioner whose role includes listening, encouraging the discussion of feelings, assimilating information through observation, assessing emotional and psychological problems, providing feedback, and reviewing options for change. He or she assists you in solving your own problems. Although the practitioner often offers guidance, clarification, and recommendations, it is *your* inner resources, strengths, and decision-making abilities that are supported in the therapy process. Psychotherapy generally progresses through a number of stages, as trust builds between you and your therapist. Some of the various techniques used by psychotherapists are described below.

*Bioenergetics* has its origins in the work of Wilhelm Reich (1897-1957), a leading Austrian psychoanalyst who supported the view that healing energy flows throughout the body and influences an individual's physical and mental well-being. He believed that chronic muscle tension works as protective armor to separate an individual from emotional pain. Alexander Lowen, a psychiatrist who studied with Reich, furthered these ideas and developed the therapeutic approach of bioenergetics, which is based on the concept that problems of the mind will physically manifest themselves in the body. If you are anxious, the body will demonstrate this emotion with increased pulse and muscle rigidity. And if your body is functioning well, your mental state will improve. Bioenergetic therapists are trained to read body language and can determine the location of physical tension resulting from repressed (pent-up) feelings. Once this area has been located, psychotherapy, physical exercises, breathing techniques, and various forms of massage can be used to release the muscle tension, increase energy flow in the body, and allow for the processing of emotions. Bioenergetics is often conducted in a group setting.

*Cognitive Behavioral Therapy* or *Cognitive Restructuring* follows the theory that negative thoughts can trap you in destructive behavior patterns, unhealthy emotions, and uncomfortable physical symptoms. For example, a student who fails a test may say, "I will never get a good report card." This thought process is a set-up for continued feelings of inadequacy. The therapist helps this student by consistently challenging the distorted thoughts and offering alternative thought possibilities that are positive, realistic, and motivating. The practitioner may reply, "What is your evidence for that? Is there another way to think about this situation? Is there anything that you can do to change that outcome?" or "This is another way to think about the situation: I received a low grade on this test. I can study next time and be better prepared. I will have a chance to improve my grades." Cognitive restructuring can result in healthier self-esteem, improved behavior, and a reduction of physical symptoms.

*Core energetics* branches off of bioenergetics. John Pierreko, a psychiatrist and body therapist, includes the element of spirituality in this body/mind technique. His theory supports that your life energy (feelings of pleasure, joy, and love) emanates from an inner core. When this energy is blocked by emotional conflict, dysfunction occurs. Using psychotherapy, bodywork (see page 41), and spiritual guidance, this technique aims to penetrate the mask of negative emotions, so that the vital energy of the core can flow freely. As a result, you are capable of being a more loving, creative, and vibrant person. Core energetics is often conducted in a group setting.

*Gestalt therapy*, a technique developed in the 1960s by Frederick Perls, concentrates on helping you become more aware of your present feelings, perceptions, conflicts, and behavior, so that you can achieve a healthy wholeness. ("Gestalt," in German, means "whole.") This approach emphasizes the expression of present feelings through dramatics. For example, you might be asked to act out the emotions related to a particular situation by using several chairs. One chair would be your shame, another would be your anger, and yet another would be your sadness. You would move from chair to chair, acting out these emotions. This dramatic exercise allows you to recognize and accept each emotional element as part of your whole being. Gestalt techniques are often conducted in group settings and offered as weekend workshops, so that results can be achieved in a concentrated period of time, rather than over many dispersed sessions.

Through *guided imagery/visualization,* you and your therapist work to find mental pictures that will stimulate natural healing responses. You may use your own imagery or work with visualizations suggested by the therapist. The images/visualizations help to alleviate anxiety and to bring about changes in attitude and behavior. They encourage you to work through emotions connected with trauma, illness, or other life circumstances. For example, a woman experiencing stage fright may imagine her fear as a rock. She pictures holding this rock in her hand and watching it turn into sand, crumbling through her fingers and disappearing. Anytime she performs in front of an audience, the woman can use this visualization to reduce anxiety and increase confidence. Therapists will often teach visualization exercises as self-help tools that you can use outside of therapy.

*Motivational Therapy* combines techniques of motivational interviewing with an understanding of the stages of change. Three psychologists, James Prochaska, John Norcross and Carlo DiClemente, became interested in how people changed and noticed that lots of people were able to change before they hit bottom. Hitting bottom means suffering severe emotional, physical and spiritual consequences before positive change is achieved. The psychologists conducted research with smokers and developed a theory called the Stages of Change. The theory names six stages of change that everyone goes through in order to change: precontemplation, contemplation, preparation, action, maintenance, and termination. The theory emphasizes that the process of change can start long before a person takes action and makes the desired change, such as losing weight, starting to exercise, or returning to school. In addition, strategies for change need to be different for people in different stages of the change process. As a result, motivational therapists will structure their therapeutic interventions based on your stage of change for your particular problem. By acknowledging your present stage of change, more productive interventions can be implemented to enhance movement towards the achievement of your personal goals.

*Neurolinguistic programming* (NLP) was developed in the 1970s by Richard Bendler, a mathematician and Gestalt therapist, and John Grinder, a professor of linguistics at Santa Cruz University. They scientifically studied leading therapists and translated the observed skills into practical techniques that could be used by other practitioners. *Neuro* refers to information that is received through the senses and from which patterns of behavior are formed. *Linguistic* pertains to the verbal and non-verbal languages, such as speech patterns and body language, that are used as tools of communication. *Programming* is a term for the set ways in which we organize our experience, behaviors, and thoughts. The goal of NLP is to reprogram negative patterns. During a counseling session, the practitioner observes your language, posture, gestures, and physiological changes (such as skin color, eye movements, and breathing). Then he or she works with you to change unconscious patterns of behavior that are negatively affecting your emotional and physical condition. Sometimes, the session includes a technique called *Using Anchors,* which may involve touch. The practitioner anchors you to a positive image by giving you a tactile cue. For example, a baseball player who has lost his ability to concentrate when getting up to bat may mentally picture the ball approaching in slow motion. The visualization is reinforced by the physical cue of rubbing his hands together. Each time he gets up to bat, the player rubs his hands and his confidence is renewed. His visualization technique enables him to make a perfect swing, thus driving the ball into the outfield. It is the use of visualization in combination with physical cues—anchors—that reinforce positive beliefs and behaviors. Visual and auditory anchors may also be used, depending on your needs. NLP achieves significant results in a short period of time and provides an empowering self-help tool.

*Stress management* helps you to cope more effectively with stress, so that the negative effects on the body, mind, and emotions can be reduced. Stress results from the normal, everyday pressures of living. Financial concerns, work obligations, and raising children are common stressors. Life-stage transitions, such as marriage, divorce, births, deaths, illness, moving, starting a new job, and unemployment, also create much anxiety and tension. Stress management training combines education on the sources and effects of stress, discussion of your particular stress reactions, and instruction in helpful coping skills. Training can take place in individual or group sessions.

During the process of psychotherapy, in addition to therapeutic dialogue, the therapist may employ techniques such as role-playing (acting out a dialogue from your life, with the therapist taking on your persona or that of a significant person), dreamwork (discussing the content of dreams), and/or journal writing (keeping a record of thoughts, feelings, or dreams). He or she may suggest that you try a new activity; interact in a different way with a friend, co-worker, child, or spouse; and/or attend a self-help meeting, workshop, or community group. This application of learning blends the accomplishments of therapy into daily life. You will then have the opportunity to process the results during ensuing therapy sessions.

The most common form of psychotherapy is individual, in which you talk one-on-one with your therapist. Other forms include couples, family, and group psychotherapy. Group sessions offer both guidance from licensed therapists and social support, offering a connection with others.

## WHAT TO EXPECT

You should expect your sessions to be held in a comfortable, professional office where privacy and confidentiality are maintained. The initial evaluation process may take one to two full sessions, during which time the therapist will ask questions about your past and present emotional state, family history, present life circumstances, experience of trauma, relationships with others, physical illnesses, medication/substance-use history, and past therapy. Before you attend your first psychotherapy session, you may find it helpful to answer the following questions: what circumstances are bringing you to psychotherapy at this time?; what do you want to change in your life or in yourself?; what do you want to get from psychotherapy?; how will you and your life be different when you achieve these changes?

When the critical problem is identified, a viable treatment plan will be formulated and discussed. The therapist should clarify fees, how often sessions will be scheduled, and the length of each session. Psychotherapy can continue for a number of years or it can be time-limited and problem-focused. In the managed care environment of today, the latter is becoming more and more common. For short-term therapy, the number of sessions is determined from the very beginning.

A psychotherapist sometimes will incorporate other alternative medicine approaches into the sessions, such as biofeedback (see page 38); flower essences (see page 55); hypnotherapy (see page 78); polarity therapy (see page 98); Reiki (see page 116); and relaxation/meditation (see page 119). Refer to the discussions on these individual approaches to learn what to expect. Even though some psychotherapy practitioners use approaches that involve light touch and/or bodywork, physical contact between a psychotherapist and a client generally is not encouraged. Aside from the occasional appropriate use of physical touch during an introductory hand shake, physical contact can confuse the professional boundary and be in conflict with the strict code of ethics that is observed by licensed psychotherapists. If you choose to combine psychotherapy and bodywork, it is recommended that you first consider seeking two separate practitioners, one for psychotherapy and a specialist for bodywork, so that clear boundaries can be maintained throughout the healing process. If your only option is to see one practitioner for both psychotherapy and bodywork, it is recommended that you participate in group sessions so that you will not feel vulnerable or isolated.

Psychotherapy can serve as a *complement* to many other approaches. For example, one goal of the energy balancing approaches— Reiki (see page 116), polarity therapy (see page 98), and Therapeutic Touch (see page 148)—is to remove energy blockages caused by physical and emotional difficulties. As energy is released, so are emotional reactions. Psychotherapy can aid in the process of coping with these overwhelming feelings and anxieties.

## COST/DURATION

*Individual: $60–$150 per session/30–90 minutes*
*Group: $15–$35 per session/60–120 minutes*

The number, frequency, and duration of therapy sessions will vary according to the specific situation. Cost depends upon the background of the therapist, the location, and your individual health plan.

## CREDENTIALS/EDUCATION

*A.C.S.W.; B.C.D.; C.S.W.; D.S.W.; L.C.S.W.; L.I.C.S.W.*
*M.S.W.; Ph.D.: Social Worker*
*D.Div.; D.Min.; M.Div.; Ph.D.: Pastoral Counselor*
*Ed.D.; M.A.; Ph.D.; Psy.D.: Psychologist*
*M.A.; M.Ed.; L.M.H.C.: Mental Health Counselor*
*M.A.; L.P.N.; R.N.: Psychiatric Nurse*
*M.D.: Psychiatrist*
*C.A.S.; C.A.D.A.C.: Substance Abuse Counselor/Addiction Specialist*

Certification and licensing of psychotherapists vary from state to state, but are generally based on academic degrees, experience, and the passing of an examination. Possible degrees and credentials for practitioners of psychotherapy are listed above. It is recommended that you seek a licensed, certified, and/or qualified psychotherapist in one of these disciplines. Please note that professionals sometimes indicate only their state certifications or licenses; they do not always refer to all of their training. (For the formal title of each degree listed above, please see *Practitioners' Credentials,* page 171.)

## HOW TO FIND A PRACTITIONER

The best way to find a psychotherapist is to contact the professional organizations listed below, which will refer you to practitioners in your area. Another method is to look in the yellow pages under "psychiatrist"; "psychologist"; "psychotherapy"; "psychiatric nurse"; "mental health counselor"; "pastoral counselor"; and/or "social worker." Also check under "health services"; "holistic/wholistic centers"; and/or "holistic/wholistic practitioners."

## PROFESSIONAL ORGANIZATIONS

American Psychiatric Association
1000 Wilson Blvd., Suite 1825
Arlington, VA 22209-3901
(888)35-PSYCH/(888) 357-7924 or (703) 907-7300
website: www.psych.org

American Psychological Association
750 First Street, NE
Washington, DC 20002-4242
(800) 374-2721 or (202) 336-5510
website: www.apa.org

National Association of Social Workers
750 First Street, NE, Suite 700
Washington, DC 20002-4241
(800) 638-8799 or (202) 408-8600
website: www.naswdc.org

## RECOMMENDED READING

Bourne, Edmund J., Ph.D. *The Anxiety & Phobia Workbook.* Oakland: New Harbinger Publications, Inc., 1995.

Rossman, Martin L., M.D. *Guided Imagery for Self-Healing.* Tiburon, CA: H.J. Kramer, 2000.

Wildermann, Ann Patterson. *Sessions: A Self-Help Guide Through Psychotherapy.* New York: The Crossroad Publishing Co., 1996.

# QIGONG

## WHAT IS IT?

Qigong exercises, consisting of meditation, relaxation, and stretching techniques, are based on the Taoist philosophy that strength is generated from within ourselves. For centuries, these techniques have been performed by individuals who are seeking to develop inner strength. Qigong is designed to avoid the tightening of muscles and the stressing of joints, and to encourage concentration on the energy flow within the body.

The ancient Chinese believed that a universal life energy—*chi*—is present in every living creature. This energy is said to circulate throughout the body along specific pathways called *meridians*. As long as chi flows freely, health is maintained. If, however, the energy current becomes blocked, the system is disrupted and pain and illness result. The goal of qigong is to develop an awareness of chi's presence and movement through techniques that bring the body into a relaxed, flexible state. Then, by strengthening and moving the essential energy of the body and enabling it to flow without obstruction, illness can be treated and health can be maintained.

## CONDITIONS THAT RESPOND BEST

Qigong is a helpful alternative medicine option for the treatment of the following conditions:

- Age-related health problems
- Anxiety
- Arthritis
- Asthma
- Back pain
- Bronchitis
- Chronic fatigue
- Chronic immune system disorders
- Concentration problems
- Constipation
- Depression
- Diabetes
- Digestive problems
- Dizziness
- Fibromyalgia
- Gastrointestinal disorders
- High blood pressure
- Insomnia
- Lack of concentration
- Low blood pressure
- Motion sickness
- Pain
- Panic attacks
- Sleeping disorders
- Stress-related disorders
- Tension headaches

This approach also aids in the achievement of the following health goals:

- General health maintenance
- Improvement of balance, coordination
- Increase in flexibility
- Increase in range of motion
- Promotion of relaxation

## HOW DOES IT WORK?

Qigong exercises involve gentle, rhythmic swinging postures, stretching movements, meditation, and deep relaxation breathing. (For further information on relaxation/meditation, see page 119.) They cultivate and move the vital energy in the body, build inner strength, and calm the emotions and the mind. The slow-paced exercises stretch every ligament and tendon, move every joint, and flex every muscle. Concentration on, and sensitivity to, the flow of the body's energy is taught through a technique that involves remaining motionless for an extended period of time (anywhere from a few minutes to an hour). The regular practice of qigong exercises leads to an improvement in circulation, balance, and flexibility, as well as an increase in range of motion. Furthermore, these exercises improve overall relaxation and awareness, and generally promote good health by encouraging a slower pace, a gentler appreciation of the body, and a clearer awareness of the self.

## WHAT TO EXPECT

You should expect a peaceful and quiet setting. Comfortable, loose-fitting clothing is recommended. Some exercises will be performed from a standing position, while others will require a sitting or reclining position. You will be performing these exercises individually. The classes are conducted in private or small group sessions, and are suitable for all ages and ranges of health.

Be prepared to let go of the burdens and stresses of your daily routine. Allow yourself to take the time to concentrate on the subtle movements of your body and the strength of your mind. The slow movements will foster a meditative state of quietness and help to clear the mind of distracting thoughts. Verbal instruction and demonstration of the various movements will be given by the instructor, but *you* are truly the practitioner of this healing art. The exercises will become more effective and more natural with practice.

## COST/DURATION

*Individual: $60 per session/45–60 minutes*
*Group: $10–$20 per session/45–60 minutes*

While feelings of relaxation and well-being are attainable from the very first class, it is recommended that you sign up for a series of qigong sessions in order to sufficiently learn proper movements and to receive the maximum benefit of this approach.

## CREDENTIALS/EDUCATION

There is presently no official certification for the practice of qigong. Those who serve as instructors of this approach have learned their skills through studies with qigong masters. It is recommended that you try one introductory class for evaluation purposes, to see if you are comfortable with the teacher and level of the course. The most important factor in selecting a qigong program is finding a positive connection with the instructor.

## HOW TO FIND A PRACTITIONER

The best way to locate a qigong instructor is to contact the professional organization listed below, which will refer you to teachers in your area. Another method is to look in the yellow pages under "qigong," "chigong," "chi kung," or "qi gung." Also check under the following headings: "health services"; "holistic/wholistic centers"; "holistic/wholistic practitioners"; and/or "tai chi." (For more information on tai chi, see page 144.)

## PROFESSIONAL ORGANIZATION

American Organization for Bodywork Therapies of Asia
   (AOBTA)
1010 Haddonfield-Berlin Road, Suite 408
Voorhees, NJ 08043-3514
(856) 782-1616
fax: (856) 782-1653
email: aobta@prodigy.net
website: www.aobta.org

## RECOMMENDED READING

Elinwood, Ellae. *The Everything T'ai Chi and Qigong Book.* Avon, MA: Adams Media Corp., 2002.

# REIKI

## WHAT IS IT?

Energy balancing approaches restore the flow of the body's natural healing energies. Such therapies typically involve various forms of light touch to relieve pain and stress and to encourage healing. Reiki (pronounced *ray-kee*) is one of these approaches. Its application is based on the belief that a universal healing energy flows around us and connects us to each other. Reiki, which means "universal life force," channels this energy into an individual's body through the hand movements of a trained practitioner. It promotes deep relaxation, stress reduction, and the release of old emotional patterns. This is a gentle, but powerful healing art that works on the four levels of an individual's being: physical, emotional, psychological, and spiritual.

Reiki is a 2,500-year-old Tibetan Buddhist practice. It was rediscovered by Dr. Mikao Usui, a Christian minister from Kyoto, Japan, in the late 1800s. Today, its techniques are passed on from masters to students. There are no religious or philosophical prerequisites associated with its use.

## CONDITIONS THAT RESPOND BEST

Reiki is an alternative medicine approach that reduces and/or relieves the following conditions:

- Addictions
- Anxiety
- Arthritis
- Asthma
- Back pain
- Balance, coordination disorders
- Chronic, debilitating illness
- Emotional problems
- Fatigue
- Immune system disorders
- Reproductive disorders
- Stress-related disorders

## HOW DOES IT WORK?

The goal of Reiki therapy is to provide physical, emotional, and spiritual healing by restoring harmony and balance to your energy field. The practitioner begins by placing his or her hands over the energy centers—often called *chakras*—of your body and sensing the present energy. Then he or she acts as a transmitter of universal life energy, receiving the energy from the environment and performing a sequence of hand movements that channel it into your body's field. Certain hand movements involve light touch on specific parts of the body. However, some practitioners do not touch the body at all; they simply place their hands very close to the targeted areas. To induce relaxation, treatment often begins on the head, and then moves to the specific part of the body that is experiencing problems.

Reiki practitioners believe that, through this approach, old energy is released and new energy flows into the body's cells. This healthy energy revitalizes and strengthens each cell, stimulating all of the body systems and normalizing functions. Thus, Reiki helps to heal illness and to prevent future disorders. In addition, it can be an effective approach for terminally ill people who are seeking to feel at peace as they move through the final stage of their lives. The balancing of energy induces a refreshing calmness and an increased sense of well-being, encouraging a healthier emotional and spiritual self.

## WHAT TO EXPECT

You should expect a comfortable, professional office where privacy and confidentiality are maintained. The atmosphere should encourage relaxation. Your Reiki treatment will be gentle and non-invasive. It will be applied to your head, your neck, the front of your torso, and on your back. You will remain fully clothed throughout the session.

During your Reiki session, you will experience a peaceful sense of warmth and well-being. It is possible that you might also experience some emotional distress at times, due to the release of repressed emotions. If these emotions seem overwhelming, it may be helpful to see a licensed psychotherapist. (See page 103 for information on psychotherapy.)

Reiki can be a powerful healing approach, and its effectiveness depends on the intuitive skill and natural healing abilities of the practitioner. He or she should be able to demonstrate a sensitive, caring, and compassionate manner for the effective transfer of healing energy. For successful treatment, be sure to select a practitioner with whom you feel absolutely comfortable.

## COST/DURATION

*$60–$80 per session/60 minutes*

It is recommended that you attend several sessions of Reiki therapy to benefit from an accumulated effect.

## CREDENTIALS/EDUCATION

*R.M.: Reiki Master*

Reiki practitioners must complete a training program with a Reiki master. There are three degrees of practice: level 1 practitioners have learned to transmit energy to themselves and others; level 2 practitioners have acquired a deeper understanding of energy transmittance; level 3 practitioners are those who become masters of Reiki therapy and teachers of others. To reach the status of master, several years of experience as a practitioner and at least one year as an apprentice to an established Reiki master must be accomplished.

## HOW TO FIND A PRACTITIONER

The best way to locate a Reiki therapist is to contact the professional organizations listed below, which will refer you to practitioners in your area. Another method is to look in the yellow pages under "Reiki"; "health services"; "holistic/wholistic centers"; and/or "holistic/wholistic practitioners."

## PROFESSIONAL ORGANIZATIONS

International Center for Reiki Training
21421 Hilltop Street, Unit #28
Southfield, MI 48034
(800) 332-8112 or (248) 948-8112
fax: (248) 948-9534

email: center@reiki.org
website: www.reiki.org

Reiki Alliance
204 N. Chestnut Street
Kellogg, ID 83837
(208) 783-3535
fax: (208) 783-4848
email: info@reikialliance.com
website: www.reikialliance.com

## RECOMMENDED READING

Barnett, Libby and Chambers, Maggie. *Reiki Energy Medicine.* Rochester, VT: Healing Arts Press, 1996.

Hunervogt, Tanmaya. *The Power of Reiki.* New York, NY: Henry Holt and Co., Inc., 1998.

# RELAXATION/MEDITATION

## WHAT IS IT?

Relaxation and meditation involve deep breathing exercises, muscle relaxation, and focused attention, all of which work toward shutting down the anxiety-producing, fight-or-flight response of the body. Some techniques also include body movements and/or exercises. Relaxation and meditation can reduce heart rate, blood pressure, breathing rate, and brain-wave patterns. The resulting state is helpful for physical and emotional healing. Many people integrate spirituality or particular religious practices into their relaxation or meditation program, as well. The psychological and spiritual benefits will vary, depending on an individual's personality, philosophy, and/or training. Some of the reported experiences include peacefulness; serenity; calmness; a sense of well-being; ecstasy or joy; selflessness; a connection to a higher being; and an altered state of consciousness. The regular practice of relaxation/meditation can decrease anxiety, alleviate symptoms of stress and disease, prevent future disorders, and provide a stronger sense of purpose and a renewed level of energy.

Throughout the history of both Eastern and Western cultures, relaxation and meditation have been practiced in a variety of ways. In the 1970s, Harvard Medical School's Dr. Herbert Benson introduced and labeled the *relaxation response*—the state of consciousness achieved through focused relaxation exercises and meditation. His pioneering work brought together many types of relaxation and meditation, from the past to the present. It became evident that even though practices and philosophies differ, the renewal processes of the body, mind, and spirit are consistently similar. One distinguishing factor is that meditation incorporates not only relaxation, but also adds a dimension of spirituality or religious/cultural tradition.

## CONDITIONS THAT RESPOND BEST

Relaxation and meditation are appropriate alternative medicine options for a variety of conditions, some of which are:

- Back pain
- Balance, coordination disorders
- Cardiovascular disorders
- Circulatory disorders
- Dermatological conditions
- Digestive disorders
- Eating disorders
- Immune system disorders
- Musculoskeletal disorders
- Nervous disorders
- Reproductive disorders
- Respiratory disorders
- Stress-related disorders
- Substance abuse
- Teeth, jaw conditions

Relaxation and meditation also can be used to achieve the following health goals:

- Anxiety reduction
- Increased energy level
- Increased sense of well-being

## HOW DOES IT WORK?

Although each person's experience with relaxation or meditation will be unique, there is a basic agenda. Secure a peaceful and quiet environment where you will not be interrupted. Next, focus on a word, sound, feeling, object, scene, or symbol. For example, visualize a pleasant landscape or contemplate a religious figure. The repetition of short words or phrases, called a *mantra*, is a very effective avenue to deep focus. The goal is to find a system that helps to clear the mind of interfering thoughts. Maintain a neutral attitude in which you can let go of distractions and not be judgmental about how well you are meditating or relaxing. Find a body position that allows you to remain comfortable throughout the process. Sitting is often suggested, but other possible positions are kneeling, squatting, sitting in the lotus position (cross-legged on the floor), or lying down. Finally, close your eyes.

With these basic principles in place, breathing techniques and muscle relaxation begin. Slow, deep breaths are encouraged as you are instructed to clear your mind and/or progressively relax different parts of your body. Through this process, you attempt to become more aware of and in control of your breathing pattern. Approximately ten to twenty minutes are needed for you to fully relax. This state is considered a unique level of consciousness that exists along the continuum between normal alertness and sleep. Some forms of relaxation/meditation also involve body movement exercises that further unite the body and the mind, and encourage the healing flow of healthy energy throughout your being. A multitude of techniques are used, some of which are discussed below.

*Autogenic training* was developed by Johannes Schultz, a German physician, in the 1930s. This technique teaches a method of relaxation in which you focus awareness on the body by repeating a series of specific phrases. These utterances affirm your ability to relieve your own muscles, and guide you through a systematic process of relaxing the entire body. For example, you would state, "My left arm is heavy," which introduces the sensation of relaxation. This phrase is repeated for every major region of the body. Then you would say, "My left arm is warm," which further relaxes the muscles, decreasing blood vessel constriction and increasing blood flow. This second clause is repeated for all major areas of the body, as well. The sequence ends with statements confirming a slow heartbeat, relaxed breathing, a cool forehead, and an overall refreshed state of mind.

*Christian meditation,* often called *contemplation,* is a process of quieting the mind with the intention of becoming more fully aware of God, the teachings of Christianity, and yourself. Prayer is used to further the meditative state. In fact, within a number of religious traditions, prayer is a form of meditation in itself, since the process of prayer generally involves taking time from normal routine to calm the mind and to focus on faith in a higher power.

*Hatha yoga* is the most common form of yoga practiced in the Western Hemisphere today. It uses stretching, breathing exercises, meditation, and classic yoga postures as ways of promoting fitness and relaxation. A yoga session will guide you through a program that improves circulation and flexibility, increases endurance, and reduces the effects of stress. (For more information on hatha yoga, see page 62.)

*Mindfulness,* a practice that stems from Buddhist meditation, is a process of being fully aware of your existence. It is a concept of staying in the present moment, without allowing outside distractions to diminish the opportunities of the immediate moment. Mindfulness helps you to become more relaxed and insightful. This technique can be used throughout the day to bring droplets of calm amidst the storm of daily life. For example, rather than rushing from the house to the car in a haze of anxiety, you can consciously slow down, take several deep, refreshing breaths, and be aware of the sky or notice a flower along the pathway. Mindfulness is used in some form throughout every relaxation and meditation practice.

*Progressive muscle relaxation* fosters awareness of muscular tension in every part of the body, and teaches methods to release that tension. It generally begins with calming breathing exercises and mental focus activities that promote serenity. Next, each individual part of the body, from the toes to the scalp, is flexed (tensed) and then released with notions of weightlessness and floating. The result is a wave of relaxation that eventually covers the entire body.

*Qigong* exercises are based on the Taoist philosophy that

strength is generated from within each person. These exercises consist of focused attention; deep breathing; gentle rhythmic, swinging postures; and stretching movements, with the intent of increasing and moving the vital energy of the body. Concentration and sensitivity to the movement of energy in the body is attained through a technique which involves remaining motionless for an allotted amount of time, ranging from a few minutes to an hour. (For more information on the qigong approach, see page 112.)

*Siddha meditation*, rooted in India, involves repeatedly reciting short words or phrases—a *mantra*. This promotes focus and relaxation. The sound helps to free the mind from distracting thoughts and provides a vibrating frequency that brings on the state of meditation. Breath control and breath awareness are also part of this technique.

*Tai chi* is a form of meditation in motion and an exercise system for which little muscular strength is required. The movements are done very slowly and have a flowing quality. By reducing the usual pace of movement, the body's habitual responses are challenged. The flowing motions exercise joints and allow energy to circulate throughout the body, dissolving chronic blocks that cause illness and discomfort. Tai chi's postures and circular movements make the body limber, help to release tension, promote relaxation, and rejuvenate the spirit. (For more information on tai chi, see page 144.)

*Transcendental meditation*, like Siddha meditation, has its origins in India and involves the use of the mantra—short words or phrases that are repeated for relaxation/meditation purposes. However, unlike Siddha meditation, the mantra is repeated in the mind, not recited aloud. This is done while sitting in a comfortable position and with your eyes closed. The goal is to achieve a deep, inner level of consciousness and relaxation.

Training in relaxation or meditation can take place in individual or group sessions. Many people enroll in local, time-limited training classes to enhance the quality of their lives. Audio tapes can be used to supplement sessions and are helpful for at-home use after your program has ended. If you participate in psychotherapy, instruction on relaxation/meditation is often incorporated into treatment (see page 119).

## WHAT TO EXPECT

You should expect a peaceful and quiet setting. You will be instructed to sit in a chair or on a floor mat; positions vary, depending on the relaxation/meditation technique and your individual preference. Comfortable, loose-fitting clothing is recommended. You will be guided through the exercises by a trained instructor, with the eventual goal of being able to perform these techniques on your own.

As mentioned above, some forms of relaxation/meditation involve physical exercises, but movements are slow and gentle. Focus is on the healthy awareness of body energy, not muscle strength and calorie burning. Therefore, the exercises will not result in soreness or discomfort. They are beneficial to all ages and body types.

Some meditation techniques are affiliated with specific religious practices or are more spiritually focused. It is important to research what will be most satisfying and effective for you. Many people find that relaxation/meditation techniques nourish body, mind, and spirit. Select a program that most adequately answers your personal needs, which may be as basic as the release of muscle tension, or as extensive as the endeavor to develop stronger insight into your spiritual self. Remember that your ability to attain a relaxed response and/or desired meditative state will improve with practice.

## COST/DURATION

*Individual: $60–$150 per session/30–90 minutes*

*Group: $15–$35 per session/60 minutes*

One relaxation/meditation session may prove effective as an introduction and can be followed-up with at-home audio tapes. In general, however, you should enroll in at least one to three group sessions, in order to learn relaxation techniques. Private instruction is often a part of psychotherapy treatment, but can be arranged as needed with a practitioner.

## CREDENTIALS/EDUCATION

For relaxation instruction, we recommend choosing a licensed psychotherapy professional with additional training in relaxation techniques. Turn to this text's section on psychotherapy for information on necessary credentials (page 111). Certification and licensing of psychotherapists will vary from state to state, but are generally based on academic degrees, experience, and examinations.

For meditation, yoga, Tai Chi, and Qigong, we recommend choosing instructors who are trained in the particular practice from reputable schools or training programs. Generally, instructors learn their skills through many years of practice with an advanced teacher. You can also consider taking an introductory class, inquiring about and checking into the instructor's credentials, and/or talking to current participants.

## HOW TO FIND A PRACTITIONER

The best way to locate a psychotherapist is to contact the professional organizations listed below, which will refer you to practitioners in your area. Be sure to indicate that you are seeking a psychotherapist with experience in relaxation training. Another method is to look in the yellow pages under "psychiatrist"; "psychologist"; "psychotherapy"; "mental health counselor"; "pastoral counselor"; "psychiatric nurse"; and/or "social worker." Other related categories include "health services"; "holistic/wholistic centers"; and/or "holistic/wholistic practitioners." In addition, relaxation workshops often are offered through adult continuing education programs, local hospitals, and health management organizations (HMOs).

To locate a meditation instructor, research the specific school or technique that is of interest to you. The below-listed organizations will provide referrals. Also, look in the yellow pages under "meditation instruction," and under the name of the specific discipline, such as "yoga" or "tai chi." (For tai chi, you can also look under "martial arts" and "self-defense.") Furthermore, check under "religious organizations" for Buddhist practices. Again, you may find "health services"; "holistic/wholistic centers"; and "holistic/wholistic practitioners" to be helpful categories.

## PROFESSIONAL ORGANIZATIONS

*Relaxation:*
American Psychiatric Association
1000 Wilson Blvd., Suite 1825
Arlington, VA 22209-3901
(888)35-PSYCH/(888) 357-7924 or (703) 907-7300
website: www.psych.org

American Psychological Association
750 First Street, NE
Washington, DC 20002-4242
(800) 374-2721 or (202) 336-5510
website: www.apa.org

National Association of Social Workers
750 First Street, NE, Suite 700
Washington, DC 20002-4241
(800) 638-8799 or (202) 408-8600
website: www.naswdc.org

*Meditation:*
American Organization for Bodywork Therapies of Asia
  (AOBTA)
1010 Haddonfield-Berlin Road, Suite 408
Voorhees, NJ 08043-3514
(856) 782-1616
fax: (856) 782-1653
email: aobta@prodigy.net
website: www.aobta.org
(for tai chi and qigong)

International Association of Yoga Therapists (IAYT)
2400A County Center Drive
Santa Rosa, CA 95403

(707) 566-9000
email: mail@iayt.org
website: www.iayt.org
(IAYT is a special division of Yoga Research and Education
    Center)

Transcendental Meditation
(888) 532-7686
(This number will ring in the state from which you are calling.
    The operator will provide you with information on
    transcendental meditation instructors near you.)

## RECOMMENDED READING

Benson, Herbert, M.D., and Eileen M. Stuart, R.N., M.S. *The Wellness Book.* New York: Fireside, 1993.

Singh, Rajinder. *Inner and Outer Peace Through Meditation.* Rockport, MA: Element, 1996.

# ROLFING

## WHAT IS IT?

Rolfing is a technique that involves deep manipulation of the connective tissue in order to restore the body's natural alignment. The practitioner performs these manipulations with the fingers, thumbs, forearms, and elbows. The agenda is to systematically treat the entire body in a series of ten sessions. Rolfing results in increased movement ability, proper postural alignment, and pain reduction.

The alignment of our bodies often can be distorted by the way we sit, stand, walk, or sleep. And as we attempt to adapt, poor posture becomes habitual. We find diminished motivation to change the patterns that eventually lead to movement restrictions and chronic pain. Ida P. Rolf (1886-1979), a biochemist from New York, believed that gravity plays a key role in healthy body structure. She theorized that if the body is properly aligned, it can work harmoniously with gravity and maintain a natural state of health and flexibility.

## CONDITIONS THAT RESPOND BEST

Rolfing is an appropriate alternative medicine option for the following conditions:

- Anxiety
- Arthritis
- Asthma
- Back problems
- Chronic pain
- Circulatory disorders
- Constipation
- Depression
- Disc problems
- Headaches
- Impaired mobility
- Indigestion
- Insomnia
- Muscle strain
- Muscular, skeletal pain
- Neck pain
- Respiratory disorders
- Sciatica
- Sore, aching joints
- Trapped nerves

This approach is also helpful in the achievement of the following health goals:

- Anxiety reduction
- Athletic performance improvement
- Balance, coordination improvement
- Postural improvement

## HOW DOES IT WORK?

The connective tissue, which joins muscles to bones and surrounds muscles, bones, and organs, is a changeable substance that constantly adjusts to the stresses placed upon the body. Physical or emotional traumas can produce a thickening of the connective tissue, resulting in restrictions of movement. With the inability of the connective tissue to function properly, the surrounding tissue takes on further responsibility. Over time, this added workload requires the body to produce greater amounts of energy, creating a loss of vitality, as well as a decrease in flexibility.

Through the use of fingers, thumbs, forearms, and elbows, Rolfing practitioners apply deep, slow pressure to soften and lengthen connective tissue, layer by layer. Each session focuses on the manipulation of the connective tissue in one area of the body. By locating and releasing the thickened areas, surrounding tissue can be restored to its proper function. During this process, the wastes and toxins that had become embedded in soft tissue are loosened and carried away. The result is increased flexibility and decreased exertion during movement.

## WHAT TO EXPECT

You should expect a comfortable, clean environment where privacy and confidentiality are maintained. The practitioner will record your complete medical history. Then he or she will focus on the physical assessment of the spinal structure, curvature, and alignment, as well as any areas of strain or tightness in the knees, legs, or feet. A photograph is often taken before the first session and after each following one, in order to show postural improvements and structural changes.

Each of the ten Rolfing sessions will last sixty to ninety minutes; they will be scheduled one week apart. Treatment will be conducted on padded treatment tables and comfortable chairs. During the session, you may experience lightheadedness due to the release of toxins into the circulatory system. However, this sensation will soon be replaced with a feeling of deep relaxation. The manipulations can be painful and some soreness may be felt after a session. Following treatment, it is recommended that you drink plenty of water and get sufficient rest. This will flush the toxins out of your system and allow for continued healing to take place.

## COST/DURATION

*$100–$150 per session/60–90 minutes*

The same fee is set for each session, and you may be given a single fee for the ten-session package. Cost varies widely, depending on the practitioner.

## CREDENTIALS/EDUCATION

*A.C.R.; C.A.R.: Advanced Certified Rolfer; Certified Advanced Rolfer*

*C.R.: Certified Rolfer*

To become a certified Rolfer, the practitioner must complete an eighteen-week training program at the Rolf Institute. A seven-week introductory course in anatomy, physiology, and kinesiology is given as a mandatory prerequisite to this program.

For the advanced certification, a Rolfer is required to have a minimum of three years experience in active practice, must take eighteen continuing education units through the Rolf Institute, and pass a six-week course at the same school. A Rolf Movement Practitioner has completed an additional four-week course.

Individuals who meet the educational requirements of the National Certification Board for Therapeutic Massage and Body-work (NCBTMB) may also sit for their exam.

## HOW TO FIND A PRACTITIONER

The best way to locate a Rolfing practitioner is to contact the professional organizations listed below, which will refer you to appropriate therapists in your area. Another method is to look in the yellow pages under "Rolfing"; "health services"; "holistic/wholistic centers"; and/or "holistic/wholistic practitioners."

## PROFESSIONAL ORGANIZATIONS

Rolf Institute
205 Canyon Boulevard
Boulder, CO 80302
(800) 530-8875 or (303) 449-5903
fax: (303) 449-5978
website: www.rolf.org

National Certification Board for Therapeutic Massage
   and Bodywork
8201 Greensboro Drive, Suite 300
McLean, VA 22102
(800) 296-0664 or (703) 610-9015
fax: (703) 610-9005
email: info@ncbtmb.com
website: www.ncbtmb.com

## RECOMMENDED READING

Bond, Mary. *Balancing Your Body: A Self-Help Approach to Rolfing Movement.* Rochester, VT: Inner Traditions Intl., Ltd., 1996.

# SHIATSU

## WHAT IS IT?

Shiatsu, a Japanese term meaning "finger pressure," is an approach that assesses and treats the body's system of energy through the application of pressure. The practice of shiatsu, which is a form of bodywork based on the principles of Traditional Chinese Medicine, dates back thousands of years. (For information on bodywork, see page 41. For a description on Traditional Chinese Medicine, turn to page 151.) Though the principles were brought to Japan from China, the techniques eventually developed into a distinct therapeutic approach. In addition to fingers and thumbs, pressure also is applied with palms, elbows, knees, and even feet. Shiatsu treats not only specific points, but also wider areas of the body. Stretches are incorporated for relaxation.

Shiatsu, like Traditional Chinese Medicine, is based on the belief that energy travels throughout the body along pathways called *meridians.* When energy flows freely through these meridians, health is maintained. However, blockages cause pain, discomfort, fatigue, and eventually lead to more serious, debilitating disorders. There are many reasons for obstructions in the energy system, including lack of exercise, poor posture, insufficient diet, and emotional stress. Shiatsu techniques actually stimulate the flow of energy, break down blockages, and restore balance.

## CONDITIONS THAT RESPOND BEST

Shiatsu is a helpful alternative medicine option for the following conditions:

- Allergies
- Anxiety
- Asthma
- Back pain

- Balance, coordination disorders
- Chronic fatigue
- Digestive disorders
- Foot and ankle pain
- Headaches, migraines
- Hormonal imbalances
- Immune system weakness
- Knee, hip, and pelvic pain
- Neck and shoulder pain
- Poor circulation
- Premenstrual syndrome (PMS)
- Restricted breathing
- Sciatica
- Sinus problems
- Skin problems
- Sleep disorders
- Stress-related disorders

## HOW DOES IT WORK?

By palpating along the abdomen, the practitioner locates energy blockages. He or she then works to release the obstructions by using sustained and stationary pressure on points along the meridian pathways and on surrounding areas. The fingers, thumbs, palms, elbows, knees, and feet can be used, depending on technique and location of treatment. During this process, wastes and toxins that previously had embedded in soft tissue are loosened and carried away. Gentle stretching and holding techniques also are used to relax the muscles. This encourages the body to remain at ease and allow for proper function.

The goal of shiatsu therapy is to balance the vital energy of the body. In doing so, this approach serves to calm the nervous system, assist the digestive process, stimulate blood flow, increase lymph circulation, and relieve muscular stiffness. Treatments tend to heighten vitality, reduce fatigue, and trigger the body's natural healing powers.

## WHAT TO EXPECT

You should expect a safe, clean environment. The practitioner will record your full medical history, addressing all relevant information, characteristics, and symptoms. He or she will conduct an examination through observation and questioning. Assessment will continue throughout the treatment. Comfortable, loose-fitting clothing is recommended. Treatment usually takes place on a floor mat. You will be lying on your back, on your stomach, on your side, and/or in a sitting position. There will be no needles, mechanical devices, or oils used.

While treatments are gentle, there may be areas that are sensitive or painful. You should maintain open communication with your practitioner, so that he or she is aware of any discomfort that you feel and can allay unnecessary concerns. During the session, you might experience lightheadedness. This is due to the presence of toxins that have been released into the circulatory system. Before long, the sensation will be replaced with a feeling of deep relaxation. The practitioner may recommend simple at-home stretching exercises to help maintain a healthy flow of energy. Dietary and lifestyle suggestions might also be recommended. It is advisable to drink plenty of water after a treatment, in order to cleanse the system.

## COST/DURATION

*$60–$120 per session/40–60 minutes*

It is advisable to attend a number of sessions, in order to benefit fully from shiatsu treatment.

## CREDENTIALS/EDUCATION

*AOBTA: American Organization for Bodywork Therapies of Asia*
*Diplomate in Asian Bodywork Therapy (NCCAOM): Diplomate in*
*    Asian Bodywork Therapy*
*Dipl. A.B.T. (NCCAOM): Diplomate in Asian Bodywork Therapy*
*NCBTMB: National Certification Board for Therapeutic Massage*
*    and Bodywork*

There is no state licensing specifically for the practice of shiatsu in the United States. However, there are some states that have Massage/Bodywork licensing laws that include Shiatsu in that category and accept the National Certification Exam for Therapeutic Massage and Bodywork (NCETMB) as part of its criteria. Further, some of these states also accept the NCCAOM (National Certification Commission for Acupuncture and Oriental Medicine) ABT (Asian Bodywork Therapy) Exam. Since licensing varies from state to state, it is recommended that you seek a practitioner who has graduated from, and been certified by, an accredited school of shiatsu. The members of the organizations that are listed at the conclusion of this section are required to meet certain professional and academic standards. A referral from these organizations will indicate that an individual has received proper training.

Practitioners who are members of the American Organization for Bodywork Therapies of Asia may use AOBTA after their names to denote that they have met the criteria necessary to join this organization. There are two levels of membership. A Certified Practitioner has had a minimum of 500 hours of training. An Associate has had a minimum of 150 hours of training. Those practitioners who have passed the ABT exam given by the NCCAOM can use either "Diplomate in Asian Bodywork Therapy (NCCAOM)" or "Dipl. A.B.T. (NCCAOM)." These practitioners have had a minimum of 500 hours of training.

## HOW TO FIND A PRACTITIONER

The best way to locate a shiatsu practitioner is to contact the professional organizations listed below to get a referral for a shiatsu practitioner in your area, or to a nearby shiatsu training institute. Many schools offer training clinics that provide treatments at reduced rates. It is important to note that qualified practitioners of shiatsu are not necessarily members of the professional organization. Another way to find a practitioner is to look in the yellow pages under "shiatsu"; "health services"; "holistic/wholistic centers"; and/or "holistic/wholistic practitioners."

## PROFESSIONAL ORGANIZATIONS

American Organization for Bodywork Therapies of Asia
   (AOBTA)
1010 Haddonfield-Berlin Road, Suite 408
Voorhees, NJ 08043-3514
(856) 782-1616
fax: (856) 782-1653
email: aobta@prodigy.net
website: www.aobta.org

National Certification Commission for Acupuncture and
  Oriental Medicine (NCCAOM)
11 Canal Center Plaza, Suite 300
Alexandria, VA 22314
(703) 548-9004
fax: (703) 548-9079
email: info@nccaom.org
website: www.nccaom.org

National Certification Board for Therapeutic Massage and
  Bodywork
8201 Greensboro Drive, Suite 300
McLean, VA 22102
(800) 296-0664 or (703) 610-9015
fax: (703) 610-9005
email: info@ncbtmb.com
website: www.ncbtmb.com

## RECOMMENDED READING

McCarty, Patrick. *The Beginner's Guide to Shiatsu: Using Japanese Finger Pressure for the Relief of Headaches, Back Pain, and Hypertension.* Garden City Park, NY: Avery Publishing Group, 1995.

Yamamoto, Shizuko, and Patrick McCarty. *The Shiatsu Handbook: A Guide to the Traditional Art of Shiatsu Acupressure.* Garden City Park, NY: Avery Publishing Group, 1996.

# SPORTS MASSAGE

## WHAT IS IT?

Touch is instinctual when it comes to providing comfort and demonstrating care. Therefore, massage—the practice of kneading or otherwise manipulating a person's muscles and other soft tissue with the intent of improving that individual's well-being—is a natural way to relax and relieve tired, sore muscles. The ancient Chinese, Greek, and Roman cultures practiced massage as part of their healing arts. Today, its therapeutic benefits continue to help many people. Sports massage is one of the numerous techniques available.

Sports massage is a form of soft-tissue mobilization that is geared toward athletes and participants of leisure sports who suffer from injuries such as major pulls, tears, strains, stiffness, pain, and/or sore spots. This type of massage is also effective for those who want to prevent the loss of mobility, enhance athletic performance, increase endurance, and maintain good health and physical conditioning. Sports massage has been used for centuries by professional and amateur athletes. It did not come to prominence in the United States until the 1970s, when well-known athletes began calling attention to the benefits of deep tissue massage before and after sporting events.

## CONDITIONS THAT RESPOND BEST

Sports massage is an appropriate alternative medicine option for the following conditions:

- Edema
- Muscle pain
- Muscle spasms
- Muscle sprain
- Muscle stiffness
- Muscle strain
- Muscle stress
- Muscle tension
- Recurring injury
- Sore spots

This approach is also helpful in the achievement of many health goals, including:

- Improvement of balance, coordination
- Improvement of circulation
- Improvement of posture
- Increase in endurance
- Increase in flexibility

## HOW DOES IT WORK?

During heavy exercise, stressed muscles develop tiny ruptures called *micro-traumas*. To protect these torn areas, the muscle cells in the injured area swell with fluid. The inflamed cells not only push painfully against nerves, but they also reduce circulation and slow the healing process. Sports massage offers a combination of techniques that breaks down scar tissue and spreads the fibers to allow for increased blood flow. Improved circulation introduces more oxygen and nutrients to the area, resulting in an accelerated healing response. During the process, inflammation decreases and fluid is carried away through the bloodstream. Lymph circulation also improves, and the wastes and toxins that previously had become embedded in the soft tissue are loosened and carried away. Sports massage includes deep stroking, deep cross fiber friction, and jostling.

In *deep stroking*, the practitioner uses his or her thumbs to apply pressure along the muscles. This technique spreads the muscle fibers, increasing blood flow to the area.

*Deep cross fiber friction* also employs thumb pressure. The practitioner works across the muscle fibers at a 90° angle with the goal of separating the muscle fibers and breaking down the adhesions that stick the fibers together.

*Jostling* is a technique during which the practitioner loosely grabs a muscle group and gently squeezes and shakes the muscles in order to relieve tension.

## WHAT TO EXPECT

You should expect a safe, clean environment that is conducive to your personal comfort. During the first visit, your sports massage therapist will record your medical history and become aware of any necessary precautions. Next, you will be asked either to lie on a well-padded treatment table or to sit in a massage chair. Comfortable clothing that allows for free movement is recommended. The therapist should be especially sensitive to draping procedures, exposing only the area of your body that requires therapeutic attention. Sports massage is usually confined to a specific area and is seldom given to the full body.

There should be clear communication between you and your therapist regarding the level of applied pressure, sensitive areas, and general comfort. Due to the fact that treatment is being applied to an injured area and that certain strokes involve rigorous movements, you may experience discomfort. However, with proper communication, your practitioner will allay any unnecessary concerns and bring you relief as soon as possible. A sports massage is generally invigorating, as tight muscles are unwound and circulation is stimulated. In order to flush the loosened toxins from your system, it is beneficial to drink plenty of water after a treatment.

If you suffer from the following conditions or situations, massage may not be an appropriate treatment, and caution is recommended: acute infectious diseases; aneurysm; bruises; cancer; fever; hematoma; hernia; high blood pressure; inflammation due to tissue damage or from bacteria; osteoporosis; phlebitis; skin conditions; varicose veins; or if you are intoxicated or on medication that contraindicates massage.

## COST/DURATION

*$60–$80 per session/30–60 minutes*

An individual session can be helpful for acute problems. If you suffer from a chronic condition, it is likely that you will require a number of treatments.

## CREDENTIALS/EDUCATION

*C.S.M.T.: Certified Sports Massage Therapist*
*NCBTMB: National Certification Board for Therapeutic Massage and Bodywork*

In order to obtain certification in sports massage, a practitioner must first complete a training program in general massage from a school accredited by the AMTA/COMTAA (American Massage Therapy Association/Commission on Massage Training Accreditation Approval) and/or the State Board of Education. The practitioner is then eligible to complete additional training from the AMTA National Sports Massage Certification Program. It is recommended that you seek a practitioner who, in addition to the above accomplishments, has passed the National Certification Examination for Therapeutic Massage and Bodywork. (For information on credentials regarding the general practice of massage, please see *Practitioners' Credentials,* page 171.)

## HOW TO FIND A PRACTITIONER

The best way to find a sports massage therapist is to contact the professional organizations listed below, which will refer you to therapists in your area or to a nearby training institute. Many massage schools offer training clinics that provide treatments at reduced rates. It is important to note that qualified practitioners of sports massage are not necessarily members of these professional organizations. Another way to locate a practitioner is to look in the yellow pages under "massage"; "sports massage"; "athletic trainers"; "health clubs"; "physical therapy clinics"; and/or "sports clinics." Ask practitioners if they specialize in the specific technique of sports massage.

## PROFESSIONAL ORGANIZATIONS

American Massage Therapy Association
820 Davis Street, Suite 100
Evanston, IL 60201
(847) 864-0123
fax: (847) 864-1178
website: www.amtamassage.org

National Certification Board for Therapeutic Massage
and Bodywork
8201 Greensboro Drive, Suite 300
McLean, VA 22102
(800) 296-0664 or (703) 610-9015
fax: (703) 610-9005
email: info@ncbtmb.com
website: www.ncbtmb.com

## RECOMMENDED READING

Benjamin Patricia J. and Lamp Scott P. *Understanding Sports Massage*. Champaign, IL: Human Kinetics, 1996.

Johnson, Joan. *The Healing Art of Sports Massage*. Emmaus, PA: Rodale Press, Inc., 1995.

# SWEDISH MASSAGE

## WHAT IS IT?

Touch is instinctual when it comes to providing comfort and demonstrating care. Therefore, massage—the practice of kneading or otherwise manipulating a person's muscles and other soft tissue with the intent of improving that individual's well-being— is a natural way to relax and relieve tired, sore muscles. The ancient Chinese, Greek, and Roman cultures practiced massage as part of their healing arts. Today, its therapeutic benefits continue to help many people. Swedish massage is the most commonly practiced massage approach of the many that are available.

Developed in Sweden during the 1800s, Swedish massage combines modern principles of anatomy and physiology with traditional Oriental practices of massage. It aims to manipulate soft tissue and muscle using the fingers and/or palms. Because Swedish massage is used widely, variations in practitioner training, technique, and length of sessions are common.

## CONDITIONS THAT RESPOND BEST

Swedish massage is a helpful treatment for the following conditions:

- Anxiety
- Arthritis
- Asthma
- Back pain
- Bronchitis
- Circulation problems
- Constipation
- Fatigue, mental and physical
- Fluid retention
- Headaches
- Heart strain
- Insomnia
- Labor and delivery pain
- Muscle pain, soreness
- Muscle spasms
- Muscle sprain
- Muscle strain
- Muscle tension
- Neck pain
- Neuralgia
- Neuritis
- Sciatica
- Shoulder pain
- Stress-related disorders
- Whiplash

This approach also aids in the achievement of many health goals, including:

- Cell nutrition
- Elimination and prevention of muscle adhesion
- Elimination of muscle waste
- Improvement of balance, coordination
- Improvement of breathing pattern
- Improvement of circulation
- Improvement of nervous system
- Improvement of posture
- Improvement of skin tone
- Increase in endurance
- Increase in flexibility
- Increase in metabolism rate
- Increase in muscle nutrition
- Promotion of relaxation
- Restoration of muscle tone
- Stimulation of kidneys
- Strengthening of joints
- Strengthening of the immune system

As the above list indicates, Swedish massage is beneficial to the health of the skeletal, muscular, circulatory, nervous, respiratory, digestive, and urinary systems.

## HOW DOES IT WORK?

Practitioners of Swedish massage perform a number of different techniques that improve circulation and release endorphins (the body's natural pain killers), including the following:

*Effleurage* involves massage strokes that glide along the skin and are applied with varying pressure. Light effleurage increases superficial blood flow to the skin, while deeper effleurage increases the flow of blood in the arteries and the movement of lymphatic fluid throughout the body.

*Petrissage* employs kneading, rolling, and gentle pinching to compress skin and muscle tissue. It increases circulation and blood flow to the muscles.

*Friction* is also a technique that compresses tissue, but differs from petrissage in that the strokes slide along the surface of the skin instead of pressing or squeezing in a stationary fashion. It is a heat-producing stroke that is useful for the breakdown of scar tissue.

*Vibration* involves quick and steady shaking motions applied with the flat of the hand or the fingertips. It can stimulate the internal organs to restore balance and trigger natural function.

*Tapotement* is a light tapping movement that serves to tone the muscles. This technique is stimulating to the nervous system.

The increase in circulation that results from a Swedish massage allows for a greater amount of oxygen to nourish the cells and aids in washing away toxins. As you heal, the endorphins decrease discomfort and provide a general sense of well-being.

## WHAT TO EXPECT

You should expect a safe, clean environment that is conducive to relaxation. During your first visit, the therapist will record your full medical history so that he or she will become aware of any necessary precautions. Then you will be asked to lie on a well-padded treatment table. Swim trunks, briefs, or gym shorts are recommended. The therapist should be especially sensitive to draping procedures, only exposing the area of the body that requires therapeutic treatment.

There should be clear communication between you and your therapist regarding the level of pressure applied, sensitive areas, and general comfort. If you have muscle strain, tightness, etc., it is likely that you will feel some discomfort until the muscles relax. However, if you keep an open dialogue with your therapist, he or she will be able to allay any unnecessary concerns and to restore well-being as soon as possible. By the end of the session, you should feel relaxed. It is beneficial to drink plenty of water after a treatment to flush the loosened toxins from your system.

If you suffer from the following conditions or situations, massage may not be an appropriate treatment, and caution is recommended: acute infectious diseases; aneurysm; bruises; cancer; fever; hematoma; hernia; high blood pressure; inflammation due to tissue damage or from bacteria; osteoporosis; phlebitis; skin conditions; varicose veins; or if you are intoxicated or on medication that contraindicates massage.

## COST/DURATION

*$60–$80 per session/30–60 minutes*

The frequency and duration of massage sessions depends on your individual preference and your condition. One session can be beneficial for relaxation and for acute problems. Chronic ailments may require a regular massage schedule.

## CREDENTIALS/EDUCATION

*C.M.P.: Certified Massage Practitioner*
*C.M.T.: Certified Massage Therapist*
*L.M.P.: Licensed Massage Practitioner*
*L.M.T.: Licensed Massage Therapist*
*M.T.; Ms.T.: Massage Therapist*
   *(does not necessarily indicate certification or licensure)*
*N.C.T.M.B.: National Certification for Therapeutic Massage*
   *and Bodywork*

The credentials of massage therapists vary from state to state, depending on licensing and certification criteria. Practitioners of Swedish massage must successfully complete program requirements from a school accredited by the AMTA/COMTAA (American Massage Therapy Association/Commission on Massage Training Accreditation, Approval) and/or the State Board of Education. It is recommended that you seek a practitioner who in addition to completing program requirements, has passed the National Certification Examination for Therapeutic Massage and Bodywork.

## HOW TO FIND A PRACTITIONER

The best way to locate a massage therapist is to contact the professional organizations listed below, which will refer you to a certified practitioner in your area or to a nearby training institute. Many massage schools offer training clinics that provide treatments at reduced rates. It is important to note that qualified massage therapists are not necessarily members of these professional organizations. Another way to locate a practitioner is to look in the yellow pages under "massage"; "health clubs"; "holistic/ wholistic centers"; "holistic/wholistic practitioners"; "physical therapy clinics"; and/or "therapeutic massage."

## PROFESSIONAL ORGANIZATIONS

American Massage Therapy Association
820 Davis Street, Suite 100
Evanston, IL 60201
(847) 864-0123
fax: (847) 864-1178
website: www.amtamassage.org

National Certification Board for Therapeutic Massage
  and Bodywork
8201 Greensboro Drive, Suite 300
McLean, VA 22102
(800) 296-0664 or (703) 610-9015
fax: (703) 610-9005
email: info@ncbtmb.com
website: www.ncbtmb.com

## RECOMMENDED READING

Mumford, Susan, *The Complete Guide to Massage: A Step by Step Approach to Total Body Relaxation.* New York: Plume (Penguin-Group), 1996.

# TAI CHI

## WHAT IS IT?

Tai chi is a form of meditation in motion and martial arts that has been practiced in China for centuries. It consists of a traditional series of slow movements that are intended to unite body and mind, build inner strength, and develop a healthy flow of life energy within the body. This exercise system requires little muscular strength, but entails much concentration and discipline. Although tai chi seems simple, it takes time to learn the proper motion and coordination. The breathing must be synchronized with the precision of the movements.

The ancient Chinese believed that a universal life energy—*chi*—is present in every living creature. Chi circulates throughout the body on specific pathways called *meridians,* allowing proper function and good health. Obstructions of this energy result in illness. Tai chi helps to create and encourage the free flow of chi. The soft-flowing movements help people of all ages to improve their physical condition, increase flexibility, decrease fatigue, and develop endurance.

## CONDITIONS THAT RESPOND BEST

Tai chi is an effective alternative medicine approach for the treatment of the following conditions:

- Anxiety
- Arthritis, rheumatism
- Asthma
- Back pain
- Bronchitis
- Chronic fatigue
- Constipation
- Diabetes
- Dizziness
- Fibromyalgia
- Gastrointestinal disorders
- High blood pressure
- Insomnia
- Low blood pressure
- Motion sickness
- Nervous disorders
- Panic attacks
- Stress-related disorders
- Ulcers

This approach can also help you to achieve many health goals, including:

- Enhancement of immune system
- Improvement of balance
- Improvement of circulation
- Improvement of concentration
- Improvement of muscle tone
- Massage of internal organs
- Strengthening of intestines
- Strengthening of spine, back

As the above list indicates, many body systems benefit from the practice of tai chi, including the circulatory, digestive, energy, gastrointestinal, immune, lymphatic, and skeletal systems.

## HOW DOES IT WORK?

Tai chi exercises are done very slowly and involve flowing motions. By moving at a decelerated pace, your body's habitual responses are challenged. As a result, you must re-evaluate every movement. This makes you more aware of the body's energy and abilities. The flowing motions cause joints to open, chronic energy blocks to dissolve, and chi to circulate throughout the body. Relaxed posture and circular movements encourage limberness, thus helping to release tension. The combination of turning, stretching, and twisting allows every part of the body to be exercised without strain. You are strengthened by the process of constant change. The slow movements of tai chi foster relaxation for the body, which encourages a meditative state in which the mind is quiet and clear of distracting thoughts. Tai chi's ability to rejuvenate, rather than exhaust, makes it a valuable exercise program in our active and fast-paced society.

## WHAT TO EXPECT

Tai chi is conducted in small groups or in private classes. You should wear clothing that allows for free movement and comfortable shoes that provide good foot support, traction, and cushioning. Beginner classes will teach basic stances, postures, and foot work. The next level will cover coordination of breathing and relaxation of movement, as well as ways to stretch and strengthen the entire body. As you progress, you will learn individual moves that are isolated and repeated several times. These are more complicated and combine the stances with upper-body movements. The final stage will involve a series of individual movements done in continuous motion. This completes the tai chi form.

Be prepared to let go of the burdens and stresses of your daily routine. Allow yourself to take this time to concentrate on the subtle movements of your body and the quiet strength of your mind. The slow movements will foster a meditative state of quietness and help to clear the mind of distracting thoughts. Verbal instruction and demonstration of the various movements will be given by the instructor, but *you* are truly the practitioner of this healing art. Expect the exercises to become more effective and natural with practice.

## COST/DURATION

*$15–$30 per class/60 minutes*

This approach is most effective when studied over a period of time, so that the movements and philosophy can become a part of your regular health maintenance.

## CREDENTIALS/EDUCATION

There is no official certification for practitioners of tai chi. Instructors are trained by tai chi masters over a number of years. It is recommended that you first try an introductory class for evaluation purposes. At that time, you can determine your reaction to the particular instructor and gather information regarding his or her experience. It is helpful to speak with students who already have been involved in the classes. The most important factor in this evaluation is your comfort level and positive connection with the instructor.

## HOW TO FIND A PRACTITIONER

The best way to find a tai chi instructor is to contact the professional organization listed below, which will refer you to teachers of this approach in your area. Another method is to look in the yellow pages under "tai chi"; "martial arts"; "self-defense"; "health services"; "holistic/wholistic centers"; and/or "holistic/wholistic practitioners."

## PROFESSIONAL ORGANIZATION

American Organization for Bodywork Therapies of Asia (AOBTA)
1010 Haddonfield-Berlin Road, Suite 408
Voorhees, NJ 08043-3514
(856) 782-1616
fax: (856) 782-1653
email: aobta@prodigy.net
website: www.aobta.org

## RECOMMENDED READING

Huang, Alfred. *Complete Tai Chi: The Definitive Guide to Physical and Emotional Self-Improvement.* Rutland, VT: Charles E. Tuttle Company, 1993.

# THERAPEUTIC TOUCH

## WHAT IS IT?

Energy balancing approaches concentrate on restoring the flow and balance of the body's natural healing energies. Such therapies typically use various forms of light touch to relieve pain and stress and to promote healing. Therapeutic Touch is one of these approaches. It is a healing practice during which the therapist uses his or her hands to direct the client's physical body energy toward healing. Therapeutic Touch is based on a philosophy that is common to much of non-Western medicine: energy flows through and around us, and any interruption in this free flow of energy leads to illness. The goal is to reprogram the body's energy so that it flows most efficiently, promoting health and preventing disease. This approach has its origins in a number of ancient healing practices, particularly the laying on of hands, which dates back to Biblical times. In the 1970s, Dolores Krieger, Ph.D., R.N., and her colleague, Dora Kunz, a spiritual healer, developed the technique that is used today.

## CONDITIONS THAT RESPOND BEST

Therapeutic Touch helps to relieve and/or reduce the discomfort of several conditions, including:

- Back pain
- Nervous disorders
- Substance abuse

This approach is also an effective alternative medicine option for the achievement of the following health goals:

- Facilitation of the body's natural restorative processes

- Promotion of relaxation and health maintenance
- Reduction of pain and anxiety
- Treatment of chronic health conditions

## HOW DOES IT WORK?

Therapeutic Touch facilitates the healing process by moving the body's energy, preventing its stagnation. Since your energy field extends beyond the surface of the skin, the Therapeutic Touch practitioner can assess this field without even touching you. He or she passes his or her hands over your body from head to toe, front to back, remaining two to four inches from your skin. The therapist may then perform rhythmical, sweeping hand motions, as if he or she is smoothing out wrinkles. Depending on the practitioner, some light touch techniques also may be used. The goal is to repattern your energy field. Therapeutic Touch can accelerate physical and emotional healing by inducing relaxation and decreasing pain through the restoration of balance within the body.

## WHAT TO EXPECT

You should expect a comfortable, professional office where privacy and confidentiality are maintained. The atmosphere should encourage relaxation. The practitioner will ask you to sit in a chair or to lie down, depending on what is most comfortable. You will not be required to disrobe. The practitioner may or may not physically touch you; it is recommended that, prior to treatment, you and your practitioner discuss the extent (or lack) of direct contact.

A state of relaxation often can be felt within the first five minutes of Therapeutic Touch therapy, and a reduction or cessation of pain symptoms can be experienced during the session. You may find it helpful to close your eyes and to clear your mind of distracting thoughts. Try to free yourself from anxieties and burdens that create tension throughout your systems. Allow yourself the time to concentrate on your body's well-being.

## COST/DURATION

*$30–$60 per session/20–30 minutes*
Response to treatment and the number of necessary sessions will

vary according to your individual needs. While one session is sometimes adequate, the treatment of chronic conditions often requires on-going therapy. Positive responses increase with the number of treatments.

## CREDENTIALS/EDUCATION

Therapeutic Touch is practiced by a variety of licensed health-care professionals. It can be used alone or in conjunction with other holistic or conventional approaches. In fact, Therapeutic Touch was specifically developed as an extension of professional skills for those in the healthcare fields. A practitioner of this approach should be a licensed healthcare professional and should have completed at least one workshop or training program on the technique. Be sure to question practitioners about their training, qualifications, and experience with Therapeutic Touch.

## HOW TO FIND A PRACTITIONER

The best way to locate a practitioner of Therapeutic Touch is to contact the professional organization listed below, which will offer referrals but does not certify or endorse specific therapists. This organization also provides information on available workshops and training. Another method to locate a Therapeutic Touch practitioner is to look in the yellow pages under "Therapeutic Touch"; "health services"; "holistic/wholistic centers"; "holistic/wholistic nurses"; and/or "holistic/wholistic practitioners." Many nurses are trained in Therapeutic Touch; contact your local hospital's nursing department and inquire if any staff nurses practice in this approach.

## PROFESSIONAL ORGANIZATION

Nurse Healers-Professional Associates International
3760 South Highland Drive, Suite 429
Salt Lake City, Utah 84106
(801) 273-3399
fax: (509) 693-3537
email: NH-PAI@Therapeutic-Touch.org
website: www.therapeutic-touch.org

## RECOMMENDED READING

Krieger, Dolores, Ph.D., R.N. *Accepting Your Power to Heal: Personal Practice of Therapeutic Touch.* Santa Fe, NM: Bear and Company, 1993.

Krieger, Dolores, Ph.D., R.N. *Therapeutic Touch Inner Workbook: Ventures in Transpersonal Healing.* Santa Fe, NM: Bear and Company, 1997.

# TRADITIONAL CHINESE MEDICINE

## WHAT IS IT?

Traditional Chinese Medicine (TCM) is a complex and sophisticated healing system. Passed down from family to family, generation to generation, its origins stem from the ancient Taoist philosophy that views the person as a whole—body and mind are unified, one influencing the other. This emphasis makes TCM one of the first holistic medicines. It is an intuitive practice that uses its own theoretical principles to identify patterns of disharmony. Acupressure (see page 11), acupuncture (see page 16), herbal remedies (see page 66), and exercise (see qigong, page 112, and tai chi, page 144) are all forms of Traditional Chinese Medicine.

The ancient Chinese believed that a universal energy—chi—is present in every living creature. Chi circulates throughout the body on specific pathways called *meridians,* allowing the body to function properly and good health to flourish. As long as energy flows freely through the meridians, health is maintained. If, however, energy becomes blocked, the system is disrupted and pain and illness result. Traditional Chinese Medicine approaches work to restore and maintain the harmony and balance of chi's flow.

The theory of *yin and yang* is foundational to the philosophy of Traditional Chinese Medicine. Yin and yang represent the principle that all aspects of life have two sides; one is no more important than the other, both work together to create harmony, and both are necessary for the experiences and processes of life. For example, we would not understand heat (yang) without cold (yin), and we would not understand light (yang) without dark (yin). The concept of yin and yang is a way of acknowledging that all things need to be viewed in relationship to one another and that everything is part of a whole. The theory also helps to explain the concept of harmony and disharmony. If you are experiencing harmony, yin and yang are equal and in balance. But excesses in one can lead to deficiencies in the other. It is this imbalance or disharmony that is targeted through the treatments of Traditional Chinese Medicine.

## CONDITIONS THAT RESPOND BEST

As mentioned above, TCM includes a number of therapeutic approaches. Each type of therapy is appropriate for a considerable list of conditions and health goals. Please refer to the specific discussion on each approach. (Page references are given at the beginning of this section.)

## HOW DOES IT WORK?

Through examination, observation, and questioning, a trained practitioner determines a pattern of disharmony. During the evaluation process, he or she addresses both physical and emotional conditions, looking not only at your outward symptoms, but also at the underlying signs that you do not immediately address. Diagnostic techniques of Traditional Chinese Medicine do not focus on finding a specific disease. Rather, your symptoms and signs are organized into a *pattern of disharmony*. This pattern becomes the basis for a treatment plan.

For example, a conventional physician dealing with a patient who is suffering from acute pain in the lower back would focus the examination on the symptom of lower back pain. Treatment might consist of bed rest, anti-inflammatory and muscle-relaxing medication, and stretching exercises. In contrast, a practitioner of Traditional Chinese Medicine who consults with the same patient may find, through examination and questioning, that the patient's back is weak, sore, and painful; the legs are without strength; and that the patient is experiencing insomnia, tinnitus, and vertigo. Furthermore, he or she is also experiencing an agitated mood; increased thirst; heavy night sweating; mild fever in the afternoon; constipation, and dark, yellow urine. The patient's tongue is red and the pulse is rapid and thin. The pattern of disharmony would be diagnosed as *deficient kidney yin.* Treatment may consist of a combination of acupuncture, acupressure, herbs, and tai chi to tone the kidneys and to increase the yin, bringing balance to the entire body.

As mentioned above, TCM prescribes a number of therapies to treat patterns of disharmony, including the following:

*Acupressure* involves the application of pressure, using fingers, thumbs, palms, and/or elbows to stimulate, disperse, and regulate the flow of energy in the body.

*Acupuncture* is an ancient method of healing in which hair-thin, disposable needles are inserted at specific points on the meridians. The stimulation serves to balance and harmonize the energy flow.

*Chinese herbalism* employs the roots, stems, flowers, and leaves of plants for a variety of medicinal purposes.

*Qigong* is a Chinese exercise system that aims to stimulate and balance the flow of chi. This approach includes low impact stretches, abdominal breathing, meditation, and visualization. (For more information on meditation and visualization, see page 119.)

*Tai chi* is a form of meditation in motion and martial arts that is based on a series of gentle exercises that are designed to unite body and mind. Slow, fluid movements are used to enhance the flow of energy while improving muscle tone and encouraging relaxation.

## WHAT TO EXPECT

You should expect to be treated in a safe, clean, and comfortable environment where privacy and confidentiality are maintained. Practitioners of TCM will be specialists in a particular area, such as acupressure, acupuncture, herbal medicine, qigong, or tai chi, which are briefly discussed above. Refer to the specific approach section for further information on what to expect. Be aware that a session may involve questions or observations that differ from Western medical practice. In order to find a pattern of disharmony, the practitioner will inquire about the functioning of the whole person, looking for underlying signs, not just the obvious symptoms. Diagnostic procedures may involve inspection of the tongue, eyes, and skin; assessment of the voice, respiration, pulse, and appearance; and questions and observations on bodily secretions and excretions (phlegm, vomit, urine, and stools); bodily odor during illness; perspiration; headaches; dizziness; pain; thirst; appetite/diet; taste and temperature preferences; sleep patterns; gynecological problems; and past and present medical history.

## COST/DURATION

*Initial Visit: $60–$225*

The above-mentioned fee gives an average cost range for the consultation visit only. Traditional Chinese Medicine is a term that refers to the use of several therapies. As a result, the duration and session cost of a regular treatment program cannot be anticipated here. Please see the specific sections on acupressure, acupuncture, herbal medicine, qigong, and tai chi for average costs and time commitments. (Page numbers are given at the beginning of this section.)

## CREDENTIALS/EDUCATION

*D.O.M./O.M.D.: Doctor of Oriental Medicine*
*M.O.M.: Master of Oriental Medicine*

The credentials listed above are for general practitioners of Oriental medicine. After an initial visit, you should be aware of which specific alternative medicine approaches will best serve your condition. The appropriate credentials and education requirements are dependent on the therapies that are suggested. For more information, please refer to the specific approach sections.

## HOW TO FIND A PRACTITIONER

The best way to find a practitioner of TCM is to contact the professional organization listed below, which will refer you to appropriate professionals in your area or to a nearby training institute for the specific approach. Many schools offer training clinics that provide treatments at reduced rates. It is important to note that qualified practitioners are not necessarily members of this organization. Another way to locate a TCM practitioner is to look in the yellow pages under "Chinese medicine/Traditional Chinese Medicine"; "Oriental medicine"; "holistic/wholistic practitioners"; "holistic/wholistic centers"; and/or "health services." Also look under the specific approach, such as "acupressure"; "acupuncture"; "herbal medicine"; "qigong"; and "tai chi."

## PROFESSIONAL ORGANIZATIONS

National Certification Commission for Acupuncture and
   Oriental Medicine (NCCAOM)
11 Canal Center Plaza, Suite 300
Alexandria, VA 22314
(703) 548-9004
fax: (703) 548-9079
email: info@nccaom.org
website: www.nccaom.org

Acupuncture and Oriental Medicine Alliance (AOMA)
6405 43rd Avenue Ct. NW, Suite B
Gig Harbor, WA 98335
(253) 851-6896
fax: (253) 851-6883
website: www.aomalliance.org

American Association of Oriental Medicine (AAOM)
5530 Wisconsin Avenue, Suite 1210
Chevy Chase, MD 20815
(888) 500-7999 or (301) 941-1064
fax: (301) 986-9313

email: info@aaom.org
website: www.aaom.org

## RECOMMENDED READING

Gascoigne, Stephen, Dr. *The Chinese Way to Health: A Self-Help Guide to Traditional Chinese Medicine.* Boston, MA: Tuttle Publishing, 1997.

# THE TRAGER APPROACH

## WHAT IS IT?

The Trager approach is a form of movement re-education consisting of a series of gentle and passive movements, along with rotation and traction of the limbs. It has no rigid procedures; movements are adjusted to the individual so that muscle tightness can be released without pain. Milton Trager, a physician from Chicago, developed the Trager approach in the early 1900s. He designed his program to help polio victims and others afflicted with neuromuscular conditions. Because of the dramatic increase in mobility that results from this treatment, even after one session, people with back pain or severe movement restrictions will find this approach most beneficial.

## CONDITIONS THAT RESPOND BEST

The Trager approach is a helpful treatment for the following conditions:

- Anxiety
- Asthma
- Back pain
- Carpal tunnel syndrome
- Cerebral palsy
- Emphysema
- Fibromyalgia
- Guillain-Barré syndrome
- High blood pressure
- Irritable bowel, spastic colon
- Migraines
- Movement restrictions
- Multiple sclerosis
- Muscular dystrophy
- Neck, shoulder pain

- Osteoarthritis
- Polio
- Sciatica
- Tendonitis
- Thoracic outlet compression syndrome

The Trager approach is also an appropriate option for the achievement of a number of health goals, including:

- Enhancement of athletic performance
- Improvement of posture
- Increase in joint mobility
- Increase in range of motion

## HOW DOES IT WORK?

You are asked to lie flat, relax, and abandon all conscious control of the body. The practitioner moves your limbs through smooth joint movements. Then, he or she gently and rhythmically rocks each part of the body, in order to communicate a sense of how light, free, and easy movement can be. As these feelings are experienced, the nerves that control muscle movement use this new information to reorganize and release patterns of tension, pain, and muscle restriction. The rocking also promotes deep relaxation, so that tension is further released on an emotional level. No force or pressure is used.

Trager practitioners are not trained to diagnose or treat specific conditions. Rather, they produce movements that deeply relax your state of mind and body. They also teach simple movements, called *mentastics,* for patients to do at home. Mentastics are designed to recreate the feelings experienced during the Trager session and to build on the benefits of the session. The effects of mentastics include an increased sense of well-being, heightened levels of energy and vitality, greater mobility, and a renewed capacity for relaxation. These benefits have been experienced by both the severely disabled and the physically fit.

## WHAT TO EXPECT

You should expect a safe, comfortable environment where privacy and confidentiality are maintained. First, the practitioner will record your full medical history. Treatment will then take place, usually on a well-padded table. You should wear loose-fitting clothing that allows for free movement. The Trager approach focuses on the trunk and limbs of the body.

During the session, the practitioner will support and move your limbs in a manner that promotes flexibility of the joints and provides pain relief. The movements are so subtle and rhythmic that you will experience the release of muscle tension without discomfort. This is a soothing and extremely effective healing approach.

## COST/DURATION

*$50–$70 per session/60–90 minutes*

Individual Trager sessions can be helpful for acute conditions. Chronic problems will benefit from repeated sessions and a commitment to at-home exercises.

## CREDENTIALS/EDUCATION

*Certified Trager® Practitioner*
*Senior Certified Trager® Practitioner*

In order to practice the Trager approach, a practitioner must complete a certification program by the professional organizations listed below, and follow-up with continuing education courses and membership renewal. Senior practitioner denotes someone who has completed 500 hours or more of training. The Trager approach is a specialty unto itself, but a variety of health professionals incorporate it into their practices.

Individuals who meet the educational requirements of the National Certification Board for Therapeutic Massage and Bodywork (NCBTMB) may also sit for their exam.

## HOW TO FIND A PRACTITIONER

The best way to locate a Trager practitioner is to contact the professional organizations listed below, which will refer you to an appropriate therapist in your area. Another method is to look in the yellow pages under "Trager"; "Trager Approach"; "health services"; "holistic/wholistic centers"; and/or "holistic/wholistic practitioners."

## PROFESSIONAL ORGANIZATIONS

Trager Institute
21 Locust Avenue
Mill Valley, CA 94941
(415) 388-2688
fax: (415) 388-2710
email: admin@trager.com
website: www.trager.com

Trager International
24800 Chagrin Blvd., Suite 205
Beachwood, Ohio 44122
(216) 896-9383
email: trager@trager.com
website: www.trager.com

National Certification Board for Therapeutic Massage
   and Bodywork
8201 Greensboro Drive, Suite 300
McLean, VA 22102
(800) 296-0664 or (703) 610-9015
fax: (703) 610-9005
email: info@ncbtmb.com
website: www.ncbtmb.com

## RECOMMENDED READING

Trager, Milton, M.D., and Cathy Hammond. *Movement as a Way to Agelessness: A Guide to Trager Mentastics.* Barrytown: Station Hill Press, 1995.

# TRIGGER POINT THERAPY

## WHAT IS IT?

Trigger point therapy, also known as myotherapy, is a bodywork technique that focuses on trigger points—tender, congested spots on muscle tissue that radiate pain to other areas of the body. (For a discussion on bodywork, see page 41.) Practitioners of trigger point therapy apply pressure to these locations, in order to relieve tension, relax muscle spasms, improve circulation, and decrease pain. The goal of this pressure is to interrupt the interior signal that is causing the trigger point and the resulting pain. Then the therapist essentially reprograms the signal through relaxing stretching exercises. Trigger point therapy can decrease the swelling and stiffness associated with neuromuscular pain, as well as increase range of motion, flexibility, and coordination.

Trigger point therapy has its origins in the work of Janet Travell, a physician from the United States who developed the procedure of trigger point injection therapy for pain and muscle problems. In the injection therapy approach, the physician locates a trigger point by palpating along the body until a tender spot is found. The trigger point is then injected with a mixture such as saline and procaine. The injections can be painful and are often followed by a gentle stretch of the area and a spray of coolant. Dr. Travell is also credited with mapping trigger points and observing how these points can radiate pain to other parts of the body. Bonnie Prudden, an American expert in the field of physical fitness and exercise therapy since the 1950s, was working with patients of trigger point injection therapy. During a treatment session in the 1970s, she applied sustained pressure to a trigger point of a client experiencing a stiff neck. The condition was relieved. From this experience, Bonnie Prudden developed trigger point therapy, which involves principles similar to trigger point injection therapy, but uses *no* injections.

## CONDITIONS THAT RESPOND BEST

Trigger point therapy is an appropriate alternative medicine treatment for the following conditions:

- Arthritis
- Bursitis
- Carpal tunnel syndrome
- Chronic back pain
- Emotional disorders
- Frozen shoulder
- Headaches
- Knee pain

- Lower back pain
- Menstrual cramps
- Multiple sclerosis
- Muscle spasms
- Muscle tension
- Muscle weakness
- Muscular pain
- Numbness
- Overuse syndromes
- Poor circulation
- Poor flexibility
- Postoperative pain
- Sciatica
- Shoulder pain
- Temporomandibular joint (TMJ) syndrome
- Tendonitis
- Whiplash

## HOW DOES IT WORK?

A trigger point can develop as a result of a fall, poor posture, or overexertion. Once established, it can be activated at any time, by physical or emotional stress. When a trigger point sends a muscle into spasm, the body responds by putting more muscles into spasm, creating a pain-spasm-pain cycle. The signals need to be interrupted in order for the body to discontinue the progression of deep, sharp, disabling muscle pain.

Trigger point therapists apply pressure directly to a trigger point for several seconds, using knuckles, fingers, or elbows. The pressure breaks the pain-signal pattern that is serving to communicate between the brain and the muscle. After the successful interruption, the muscle relaxes and is then passively stretched. The neuromuscular system (which includes nerves that control muscle function) uses this new information to reorganize, thus relieving tension, pain, and restriction. In addition, a series of exercises are introduced to keep the muscle pain-free. These exercises gently develop healthy function. Clients are taught to avoid pain-producing posture and to stretch and strengthen muscles, so that they can avoid the recurrence of trigger points.

## WHAT TO EXPECT

You should expect a safe, clean environment. The practitioner will begin with a series of questions, in order to determine the cause and area of your discomfort. Depending on the location of your pain, sessions will be performed on a padded treatment table or in a treatment chair. It is recommended that you wear a swimsuit or comfortable, loose-fitting clothing that allows for free movement.

To locate a trigger point, the therapist will press along a muscle. This process can be painful, but with good dialogue between you and your therapist, it can be brief. Clear communication should always be maintained regarding the level of pain and the amount of pressure applied. As the practitioner works, he or she will ask you to describe the level of pain. Once a trigger point is found, the therapist will apply pressure for several seconds and then slowly release. You can expect to feel relief immediately after the applied pressure. The practitioner will also stretch the muscle being treated, and may instruct you on exercises to be done at home.

## COST/DURATION

*$45–$80 per session/30–60 minutes*

Some acute problems can be relieved in one session. Chronic problems generally require repeated treatments, even considering the at-home exercises.

## CREDENTIALS/EDUCATION

*C.B.P.M.: Certified Bonnie Prudden Myotherapist*

Practitioners of trigger point therapy should be certified with the above credential, which involves a nine-month, 1,400-hour training program, a board examination, and forty-five hours of continuing education units every other year. Trigger point therapy is an independent field, but various healthcare practitioners incorporate this approach into their work.

## HOW TO FIND A PRACTITIONER

The best way to find a trigger point therapist is to contact the professional organization listed below, which will refer you to certified practitioners in your area. Another method is to look in the yellow pages under "health services"; "holistic/wholistic centers"; "holistic/wholistic practitioners"; "myotherapy"; and/ or "trigger point therapy."

## PROFESSIONAL ORGANIZATIONS

Bonnie Prudden Myotherapy
4330 East Havasu Road
Tucson, AZ 85718
(800) 221-4634 or (520) 529-3979
fax: (520) 529-6679
www.bonnieprudden.com

International Myotherapy Association
email: info@myotherapy.org
website: www.myotherapy.org

## RECOMMENDED READING

Prudden, Bonnie. *Pain Erasure: The Bonnie Prudden Way.* New York: Ballantine Books, 1985.

# Glossary

**acute illness.** A physical or emotional condition that has a rapid onset requiring immediate attention.

**alternative medicine.** A term used to describe holistic/wholistic healing approaches that support and work in partnership with conventional medicine.

**approach.** A general term referring to any alternative medicine treatment method.

**balance.** Refers to the state in which the body and mind have equal influence on a person's health and are operating optimally to maintain health; the equality between body and mind.

**bodywork.** Refers to a number of therapeutic approaches that involve manipulation and the balancing of the musculoskeletal system to facilitate healing, relieve pain, increase energy, and promote relaxation and well-being. Bodywork approaches use hands-on techniques.

**cardiovascular training.** Physical conditioning that strengthens the heart and blood vessels.

**central nervous system (CNS).** This system, which consists of the brain and the spinal cord, controls and coordinates much of the body's functioning.

**cerebrospinal fluid.** The clear fluid that circulates through and around the brain and spinal cord.

**chakras.** The spiritual energy centers of the body.

**chi.** A traditional Chinese medical term for the healing energy/universal life energy that circulates throughout the body.

**chronic illness.** A long-term physical or emotional condition, usually with a slow-developing onset, often lasting for life, that is either persistently active or reoccurs frequently.

**circulatory system.** This system, which includes the heart and the blood vessels, is responsible for the continuous flow of blood throughout the body.

**complementary care.** A term used to describe holistic/wholistic healing approaches that support and work in partnership with conventional medicine.

**detoxification.** The process of breaking down and eliminating poisonous substances in the body.

**dilution.** In homeopathic care, the process of adding water or alcohol to a remedy. Dilution ultimately strengthens the remedy because its healing potential increases as the amount of the symptom-producing substance decreases.

**disharmony.** Refers to the interruption of the smooth interaction of body systems.

**dosha.** According to Ayurvedic medicine, a basic operating principle necessary for the body's healthy functioning. There are three doshas: kapha, pitta, and vata.

**draping.** The appropriate use of linens to avoid unnecessary exposure, to keep a client covered, during bodywork.

**dysfunction.** Abnormal or unhealthy functioning; refers to the interruption of the smooth interaction of body systems.

**endocrine system.** A system of glands in the body that releases hormones into the bloodstream.

**endorphin.** A brain chemical that serves as the body's natural opiate or pain killer.

**energy.** A vital life force that surrounds and flows through the body.

**energy balancing.** Restoring the flow and balance of the body's natural healing energies. Energy balancing approaches use various forms of light touch to relieve pain and stress and to promote healing.

**function.** In the holistic/wholistic context, this term describes for what an herb is used. For example, ginger's *function* is to remedy a dry, sore throat.

**guided imagery.** Also referred to as *visualization*, this is a process that aims to facilitate healing through the creation of calming images or scenes in the mind. This technique is used as a method of relaxation, helping to alleviate anxiety and to bring about changes in attitude and behavior.

**harmony.** Refers to the smooth interaction of systems in the body and mind.

**holistic health.** A philosophy of healing that takes into consideration aspects of the whole person; physical, emotional, mental, spiritual, social, and environmental factors are addressed. Holistic (or wholistic) health emphasizes the individual's active involvement in his or her own healthcare.

**hydrotherapy.** The application of water in its various forms (liquid, solid, vapor) for therapeutic purposes, often used as an adjunct treatment, especially to massage.

**immune system.** A combination of body systems that works toward fighting bacteria and other foreign substances.

**iridology.** A diagnostic approach used to clarify the underlying cause of a disease through eye assessment.

**kapha.** According to Ayurvedic medicine, the dosha that is responsible for the structure of the body and includes muscles, fat, and bones. Also, the body type (prakriti) that includes, among others, the following characteristics: heavy build, slow-functioning systems, and a relaxed nature that expresses both sympathy and stubbornness.

**kneading.** Used with bodywork approaches, this hands-on technique consists of lifting, squeezing and pressing the soft tissue of the body.

**Law of Potentization.** One of the primary principles of homeopathic medicine, this law states that the smaller the dose of a homeopathic remedy, and the more it is diluted and shaken, the greater its potency and effect in combating an illness.

**Law of Similars.** This ancient law states that a disease is cured by the application of remedies that produce symptoms similar to those of the disease.

**laying on of hands.** An ancient therapeutic approach, used in many forms of energy work and massage, in which hands are placed upon an individual to generate healing energy.

**lymph.** A body fluid that functions to remove foreign matter from the cell environment, transport necessary substances, and restore proper fluid content.

**lymph nodes.** Small organs in the lymphatic vessels that filter foreign matter from the body, combat infection, and serve as sites for the production of white blood cells and blood plasma cells.

**lymphatic system.** This system consists of the lymphatic vessels, lymph nodes, tonsils, spleen, and thymus. It makes, filters, and circulates lymph.

**manipulation.** The movement and adjustment of the joints and soft tissue of the body.

**mantra.** Short words or phrases that are repeatedly recited (verbally or mentally) for meditative/relaxation purposes.

**meninges.** The membranes that surround the brain and spinal cord.

**mercury amalgam.** An alloy (a mixture of two or more metals) of mercury and other metals used by dentists to fill cavities in the teeth. This substance is suspected of endangering health.

**meridians.** The pathways through which the healing energy (chi) of the body flows.

**metabolism.** The chemical processes of the body that break down and synthesize substances for energy, nutrition, growth, waste-release, and other activities for the maintenance of life.

**moxa.** A Chinese herb that is burned on or near the body to strengthen and move healing energy (chi). Moxa is also known as mugwort, or *Artemisia vulgaris.*

**moxibustion.** The act of burning moxa on or near the body to strengthen and move its healing energy (chi).

**neuromuscular system.** This term refers to the nerves and muscles of the body.

**neurotransmitters.** Chemicals that help to carry nerve impulses between nerve cells.

**organic foods.** Foods that are grown without pesticides, herbicides, or other synthetic chemicals.

**osteopathy.** A branch of medicine that primarily uses manipulation therapy to restore the body structure to optimal mobility and flexibility, resulting in pain relief and overall health improvement.

**passive movement.** The gentle movement of a patient's limb by a practitioner, without the active involvement of the patient.

**pitta.** According to Ayurvedic medicine, the dosha that is responsible for processing nutrients, air, and water in the body Also, the body type (prakriti) that includes, among others, the following characteristics: medium size, fervent, intelligent, with a strict regularity of mind and body.

**plaque.** A filmy substance, consisting of mucus and bacteria, that accumulates on the tooth surface and can lead to tooth decay.

**potentization.** In homeopathic care, the process of shaking a remedy in order to agitate the molecules, thus activating the medication.

**prakriti.** The Sanskrit word for "nature"; refers to body type, as assigned by Ayurvedic medicine. There are three prakritis: kapha, pitta, and vata.

**property.** In the holistic/wholistic context, this term refers to how an herb works. For example, ginger has the *property* of a stimulant that activates the salivary glands.

**psychotic.** A person afflicted with the severe mental illness of psychosis, indicated primarily by a loss of contact with reality, bizarre behavior, hallucinations, and/or delusions.

**range of motion.** The movement of joints in the body from their original position to their full extension.

**rasayana.** Herbs and minerals used to promote longevity. They are sold in the United States as herbal food supplements.

**regression.** A return to child-like behavior or early life experiences.

**repression.** A defense mechanism that involves pushing painful experiences and feelings into the unconscious mind and out of conscious awareness.

**respiratory system.** This system delivers oxygen to the cells of the body and carries away carbon dioxide waste.

**soft tissue.** Consists of the muscles, tendons, ligaments, and organs of the body.

**stagnation.** A blockage of healing energy (chi) in the meridian pathways of the body.

**Taoism.** A Chinese religious philosophy from the 6th Century B.C., based on the teachings of Lao-Tse.

**toxins.** Poisonous substances.

**trance.** A sleep-like state in which an individual mentally detaches from his or her physical environment and conscious mind. Hypnosis induces a trance-like state.

**vata.** According to Ayurvedic medicine, the dosha that is responsible for respiration, blood circulation, digestion, and nervous system functioning. Also, the body type (prakriti) that includes, among others, the following characteristics: slim, nervous, very energetic, and erratic in behavior and body systems.

**visualization.** Also referred to as *guided imagery,* this is a process that aims to facilitate healing through the creation of calming images or scenes in the mind. This technique is used as a method of relaxation, helping to alleviate anxiety and to bring about changes in attitude and behavior.

**vitality.** The underlying strength and energy that allows you and your body to function.

**weight training.** The use of weights during exercise training to increase strength, tone the muscles, and improve circulation.

**wellness.** A state of good health of the body, mind, and spirit.

**wholistic health.** A philosophy of healing that takes into consideration aspects of the whole person; physical, emotional, mental, spiritual, social, and environmental factors are addressed. Wholistic (or holistic) health emphasizes the individual's active involvement in his or her own health care.

**yin and yang.** This concept comes from ancient Chinese medicine and represents the idea that all things are comprised of two opposite components, such as hot and cold or light and dark. It is a belief of interdependence; one component cannot exist without the other. The human system needs both yin and yang for balance.

# Practitioners' Credentials

When seeking a practitioner of a specific approach, it is important to familiarize yourself with the degrees, certifications, licenses, etc. that are suggested and/or required for practice. A list of such credentials for the approaches discussed in this book is given below. There are no mandatory requirements or state regulations for the approaches that are not listed. Refer to the individual sections for more information.

Please be aware that there is a difference between being *certified* and being *licensed*. For example, *C.M.T. or* C.M.P. (certified massage therapist or certified massage practitioner, respectively) indicates a massage therapist who has been certified by virtue of having graduated from an accredited school of therapeutic massage. *L.M.T. or* L.M.P. (licensed massage therapist or licensed massage practitioner, respectively) indicates that in addition to having graduated from an accredited school of therapeutic massage, the practitioner has met the licensing requirements of a particular state. It is important to note that licensing is not available in all states. For example, in Massachusetts, massage therapists are certified only, since licensing is not presently available at the state level.

**Acupressure:**
AOBTA: American Organization for Bodywork Therapies of Asia
Dipl. A.B.T. (NCCAOM): Diplomate in Asian Bodywork Therapy

Diplomate in Asian Bodywork Therapy (NCCAOM): Diplomate in Asian Bodywork Therapy
NCBTMB: National Certification Board for Therapeutic Massage and Bodywork

**Acupuncture:**
C.A.: Certified Acupuncturist
Dipl.Ac. (NCCAOM): Diplomate
 in Acupuncture
Diplomate in Acupuncture
 (NCCAOM): Diplomate in
 Acupuncture
L.Ac.Lic.Ac.: Licensed
 Acupuncturist
M.Ac.: Master of Acupuncture
R.Ac.: Registered Acupuncturist

**Alexander Technique:**
AmSAT: American Society of the
 Alexander Technique

**Aquatic Therapy:**
Certified Aquatic Exercise
 Instructor
CPR and First Aid (certification)
W.S.I.: Water Safety Instructor
 (Red Cross certification)

**Aromatherapy:**
NAHA: National Association for
 Holistic Aromatherapy
RA™: Registered Aromatherapist

**Ayurveda:**
B.A.M.S.: Bachelor of Ayurveda
 Medical Studies

**Biofeedback:**
B.C.I.A.C.: Biofeedback
 Certification Institute of
 America Certified

**Chiropractic:**
D.C.: Doctor of Chiropractic

**CranioSacral Therapy:**
C.S.T.: CranioSacral Therapist
IAHP: International Association
 of Healthcare Practitioners

**Feldenkrais Method:**
G.C.F.P.: Guild Certified
 Feldenkrais Practitioner

*FGNA practitioners may also use
the following service marked terms:*
Awareness Through Movement®
Feldenkrais®
Feldenkrais Method®
Functional Integration®
Guild Certified Feldenkrais
 Practitioner℠
Guild Certified Feldenkrais
 Teacher℠

**Foot Reflexology:**
Certified in the Original Ingham
 Method
NCBTMB: National Certification
 Board for Therapeutic Massage
 and Bodywork

**Herbal Medicine:**
Diplomate in Chinese Herbology
 (NCCAOM)
Dipl. C.H. (NCCAOM)

**Holistic Dentistry:**
D.D.S.: Doctor of Dental Surgery
D.M.D.: Doctor of Medical
 Dentistry

**Homeopathy:**
C.C.H.: Certified in Classical
 Homeopathy

D.Ht.: Diplomate in Homeotherapeutics

D.H.A.N.P.: Diplomate in Homeopathic Academy of Naturopathic Physicians

**Hypnotherapy:**
C.H.: Certified Hypnotherapist

**Lymphatic Massage:**
C.M.L.D.T.: Certified Manual Lymph Drainage Therapist

IAHP: International Association of Healthcare Professionals

*For massage, in general:*
C.M.P.; C.M.T.: Certified Massage Practitioner; Certified Massage Therapist

L.M.P.; L.M.T.: Licensed Massage Practitioner; Licensed Massage Therapist

M.T./Ms.T.: Massage Therapist (does not necessarily indicate certification or licensure)

NCBTMB: National Certification Board for Therapeutic Massage and Bodywork

**Naturopathy:**
N.D.: Doctor of Naturopathic Medicine

**Nutritional Counseling:**
C.N.C.®: Certified Nutritional Consultant

L.D.: Licensed Dietitian

R.D.: Registered Dietitian

**Polarity Therapy:**
R.P.P.: Registered Polarity Practitioner

NCBTMB: National Certification Board for Therapeutic Massage and Bodywork

**Psychotherapy:**

*Mental Health Counselor:*
M.A.: Master of Arts
M.Ed.: Master of Education

*Psychiatrist:*
M.D.: Medical Doctor

*Psychologist:*
Ed.D.: Doctor of Education
M.A.: Master of Arts
Ph.D.: Doctor of Philosophy
Psy.D.: Doctor of Psychology

*Social Worker:*
A.C.S.W.: Academy of Certified Social Workers
B.C.D.: Board Certified Diplomate in Clinical Social Work
C.S.W.: Certified Social Worker
D.S.W.: Doctor of Social Work
L.C.S.W.: Licensed Clinical Social Worker
L.I.C.S.W.: Licensed Independent Clinical Social Worker
M.S.W.: Master of Social Work
Ph.D.: Doctor of Philosophy

*Pastoral Counselor:*
D.Div.: Doctor of Divinity
D.Min.: Doctor of Ministry
M.Div.: Master of Divinity
Ph.D.: Doctor of Philosophy

*Psychiatric Nurse:*
M.A.: Master of Arts
R.N.: Registered Nurse

**Reiki:**
R.M.: Reiki Master

**Rolfing:**
A.C.R.; C.A.R.: Advanced
Certified Rolfer; Certified
Advanced Rolfer
C.R.: Certified Rolfer
NCBTMB: National Certification
Board for Therapeutic Massage
and Bodywork

**Shiatsu:**
AOBTA: American Organization
for Bodywork Therapies of
Asia
Diplomate in Asian Bodywork
Therapy (NCCAOM):
Diplomate in Asian
Bodywork Therapy
Dipl. A.B.T. (NCCAOM):
Diplomate in Asian
Bodywork Therapy
NCBTMB: National Certification
Board for Therapeutic Massage
and Bodywork

**Sports Massage:**
C.S.M.T.: Certified Sports
Massage Therapist
NCBTMB: National Certification
Board for Therapeutic Massage
and Bodywork

*For massage, in general:*
C.M.P.; C.M.T.: Certified Massage
Practitioner; Certified Massage
Therapist

L.M.P.; L.M.T.: Licensed Massage
Practitioner; Licensed Massage
Therapist
M.T./Ms.T.: Massage Therapist
(does not necessarily indicate
certification or licensure)

**Swedish Massage:**
C.M.P.; C.M.T.: Certified Massage
Practitioner; Certified Massage
Therapist
L.M.P.; L.M.T.: Licensed Massage
Practitioner; Licensed Massage
Therapist
M.T./Ms.T.: Massage Therapist
(does not necessarily indicate
certification or licensure)
NCBTMB: National Certification
Board for Therapeutic Massage
and Bodywork

**Traditional Chinese
Medicine:**
D.O.M./O.M.D.: Doctor of
Oriental Medicine
M.O.M.: Master of Oriental
Medicine

**Trager Approach:**
C.T.P.: Certified Trager
Practitioner
NCBTMB: National Certification
Board for Therapeutic Massage
and Bodywork

**Trigger Point Therapy:**
C.B.P.M.: Certified Bonnie
Prudden Myotherapist

# Professional Organizations

Professional organizations and teaching institutions that can forward further information and/or refer you to a practitioner in your area are listed below.

**Acupressure:**

American Organization for Bodywork Therapies of Asia (AOBTA)
1010 Haddonfield-Berlin Road, Suite 408
Voorhees, NJ 08043-3514
(856) 782-1616
fax: (856) 782-1653
email: aobta@prodigy.net
website: www.aobta.org

National Certification Commission for Acupuncture and Oriental Medicine (NCCAOM)
11 Canal Center Plaza, Suite 300
Alexandria, VA 22314
(703) 548-9004
fax: (703) 548-9079
email: info@nccaom.org
website: www.nccaom.org

National Certification Board for Therapeutic Massage and Bodywork
8201 Greensboro Drive, Suite 300
McLean, VA 22102
(800) 296-0664 or (703) 610-9015
email: info@ncbtmb.com
website: www.ncbtmb.com

**Acupuncture:**

National Certification Commission for Acupuncture and Oriental Medicine (NCCAOM)
11 Canal Center Plaza, Suite 300
Alexandria, VA 22314
(703) 548-9004
fax: (703) 548-9079
email: info@nccaom.org
website: www.nccaom.org

Acupuncture and Oriental Medicine Alliance (AOMA)
6405 43rd Avenue Ct. NW, Suite B
Gig Harbor, WA 98335
(253) 851-6896
fax: (253) 851-6883
website: www.aomalliance.org

## The Alexander Technique:
American Society of the
  Alexander Technique (AmSAT)
P.O. Box 60008
Florence, MA 01062
(800) 473-0620
fax: (413) 584-3097
website: www.alexandertech.org

## Aquatic Therapy:
Aquatic Exercise Association
3439 Technology Drive, Unit 6
Nokomis, FL 34274-3627
(941) 486-8600 or
  (888) AEA-WAVE/888-232-9283
fax: (941) 486-8820
email: info@aeawave.com
website: www.aeawave.com

Red Cross (local chapters found
  in your yellow pages)

## Aromatherapy:
National Association for Holistic
  Aromatherapy (NAHA)
4509 Interlake Avenue N., #233
Seattle, WA 98103-6773
(888) ASK-NAHA/(888) 275-6242
  or (206) 547-2164
fax: (206) 547-2680
email: info@naha.org
website: www.naha.org

Aromatherapy Registration
  Council (ARC)
email:
  info@aromatherapycouncil.org
website: www.aromatherapy
  council.org (you can download
  a register of Registered
  Aromatherapists™)

## Ayurvedic Medicine:
The Ayurvedic Institute
P.O. Box 23445
Albuquerque, NM 87192-1445
(505) 291-9698
fax: (505) 294-7572
website: www.ayurveda.com

## Biofeedback:
Biofeedback Certification
  Institute of America (BCIA)
10200 W. 44th Avenue,
  Suite 310
Wheat Ridge, CO 80033-2840
(303) 420-2902
fax: (303) 422-8894
email: bcia@resourcenter.com
website: www.bcia.org

Association for Applied
  Psychophysiology and
  Biofeedback (AAPB)
10200 W. 44th Avenue, Suite 304
Wheat Ridge, CO 80033-2840
(303) 422-8436
fax: (303) 422-8894
email: aapb@resourcenter.com
website: www.aapb.org
*The AAPB does not certify
  practitioners, it is geared
  towards research in the field.

## Chiropractic:
American Chiropractic
  Association (ACA)
1701 Clarendon Boulevard
Arlington, VA 22209
(800) 986-4636
fax: (703) 243-2593
website: www.amerchiro.org

## CranioSacral Therapy:
International Association of
   Healthcare Practitioners
   (IAHP)
11211 Prosperity Farms Road,
   Suite D-325
Palm Beach Gardens, FL
   33410-3487
(800) 311-9204 or (561) 622-4334
fax: (561) 622-4771
email: iahp@iahp.com
website: www.iahp.com

## The Feldenkrais Method:
Feldenkrais Guild® of North
   America (FGNA)
3611 SW Hood Avenue,
   Suite 100
Portland, OR 97201
(800) 775-2118 or (503) 221-6612
fax: (503) 221-6616
website: www.feldenkrais.com

## Flower Essences:
Flower Essence Society (FES)
P.O. Box 459
Nevada City, CA 95959
(800) 736-9222 or (530) 265-9163
fax: (530) 265-0584
email: mail@flowersociety.org
website: www.flowersociety.org

Nelson Bach USA
Educational Programs
100 Research Drive
Wilmington, MA 01887
(800) 334-0843 or (978) 988-3833
fax: (978) 988-0233
email: education@nelsonbach.com
website: www.nelsonbach.com

## Foot Reflexology:
International Institute of
   Reflexology, Inc.
5650 First Avenue, North
P.O. Box 12642
St. Petersburg, FL 33733-2642
(727) 343-4811
fax: (727) 381-2807
email: iir@tampabay.rr.com
website: www.reflexology-usa.net

## Hatha Yoga:
International Association of Yoga
   Therapists (IAYT)
2400A County Center Drive
Santa Rosa, CA 95403
(707) 566-9000
email: mail@iayt.org
website: www.iayt.org
(IAYT is a special division of Yoga
   Research and Education Center)

## Herbal Medicine:
American Holistic Medical
   Association (AHMA)
12101 Menaul Blvd. N.E., Suite C
Albuquerque, NM 87112
(505) 292-7788
fax: (505) 293-7582
email: info@holisticmedicine.org
website:
   www.holisticmedicine.org

Acupuncture and Oriental
   Medicine Alliance
6405 43rd Avenue Ct. NW, Suite B
Gig Harbor, WA 98335
(253) 851-6896
fax: (253) 851-6883
website: www.aomalliance.org

National Certification
 Commission for Acupuncture
 and Oriental Medicine
 (NCCAOM)
11 Canal Center Plaza, Suite 300
Alexandria, VA 22314
(703) 548-9004
fax: (703) 548-9079
email: info@nccaom.org
website: www.nccaom.org

**Holistic Dentistry:**
Foundation for Toxic Free
 Dentistry (FTFD)
P.O. Box 608010
Orlando, FL 32860-8010
(send a 78-cent #10 SASE for
 information on holistic
 dentists)

**Homeopathy:**
National Center for Homeopathy
801 N. Fairfax Street, Suite 306
Alexandria, VA 22314
(877) 624-0613 or (703) 548-7790
fax: (703) 548-7792
email: info@homeopathic.org
website: www.homeopathic.org

**Hypnotherapy:**
American Board of
 Hypnotherapy
2002 E. McFadden Avenue,
 Suite 100
Santa Ana, CA 92705
(800) 872-9996 or (714) 245-9340
fax: (714) 245-9881
email: info@hypnosis.com
website: www.hypnosis.com

The American Society of Clinical
 Hypnosis
140 N. Bloomingdale Road
Bloomingdale, IL 60108-1017
(630) 980-4740
fax: (630) 351-8490
email: info@asch.net
website: www.asch.net

International Medical and Dental
 Hypnotherapy Association
4110 Edgeland, Suite 800
Royal Oak, MI 48073-2285
(248) 549-5594 or (800) 257-5467
website: www.infinityinst.com

National Guild of Hypnotists
P.O. Box 308
Merrimack, NH 03054-0308
(603) 429-9438
fax: (603) 424-8066
email: ngh@ngh.net
website: www.ngh.net

**Lymphatic Massage:**
North American Vodder
 Association of Lymphatic
 Therapy
356 Waterbury Drive
East Lake, OH 44095
(888) 462-8258
website: www.navalt.com

International Association of
 Healthcare Practitioners (IAHP)
11211 Prosperity Farms Road,
 Suite D-325
Palm Beach Gardens, FL
 33410-3487

(800) 311-9204 or (561) 622-4334
fax: (561) 622-4771
email: iahp@iahp.com
website: www.iahp.com

## Naturopathy:

The American Association of
  Naturopathic Physicians
3201 New Mexico Avenue NW,
  Suite 350
Washington, DC 20016
(866) 538-2267 or (202) 895-1392
fax: (202) 274-1992
website: www.naturopathic.org

## Nutritional Counseling:

The American Association of
  Naturopathic Physicians
3201 New Mexico Avenue NW,
  Suite 350
Washington, DC 20016
(866) 538-2267 or (202) 895-1392
fax: (202) 274-1992
website: www.naturopathic.org

American Association of
  Nutritional Consultants
400 Oak Hill Drive
Winona Lake, IN 46590
(888) 828-2262
fax: (574) 269-4060
email: registrar@aanc.net
website: www.aanc.net

American Dietetic Association
120 South Riverside Plaza,
  Suite 2000
Chicago, IL 60606-6995
(800) 877-1600 or (312) 899-0040
Website: www.eatright.org

The Ayurvedic Institute
P.O. Box 23445
Albuquerque, NM 87192-1445
(505) 291-9698
fax: (505) 294-7572
website: www.ayurveda.com

Acupuncture and Oriental
  Medicine Alliance (AOMA)
6405 43rd Avenue Ct. NW, Suite B
Gig Harbor, WA 98335
(253) 851-6896
fax: (253) 851-6883
website: www.aomalliance.org

## Polarity Therapy:

American Polarity Therapy
  Association
P.O. Box 19858
Boulder, CO 80308
(303) 545-2080
fax: (303) 545-2161
email: hq@polaritytherapy.org
website:
  www.polaritytherapy.org

National Certification Board for
  Therapeutic Massage and
  Bodywork
8201 Greensboro Drive, Suite 300
McLean, VA 22102
(800) 296-0664 or (703) 610-9015
fax: (703) 610-9005
email: info@ncbtmb.com
website: www.ncbtmb.com

## Psychotherapy:

American Psychiatric Association
1000 Wilson Blvd., Suite 1825
Arlington, VA 22209-3901

(888)35-PSYCH/(888) 357-7924
or (703) 907-7300
website: www.psych.org

American Psychological
   Association
750 First Street, NE
Washington, DC 20002-4242
(800) 374-2721 or (202) 336-5510
website: www.apa.org

National Association of Social
   Workers
750 First Street, NE, Suite 700
Washington, DC 20002-4241
(800) 638-8799 or (202) 408-8600
website: www.naswdc.org

## Qigong:
American Organization for
   Bodywork Therapies of Asia
   (AOBTA)
1010 Haddonfield-Berlin Road,
   Suite 408
Voorhees, NJ 08043-3514
(856) 782-1616
fax: (856) 782-1653
email: aobta@prodigy.net
website: www.aobta.org

## Reiki:
International Center for Reiki
   Training
21421 Hilltop Street, Unit #28
Southfield, MI 48034
(800) 332-8112 or (248) 948-8112
fax: (248) 948-9534
email: center@reiki.org
website: www.reiki.org

Reiki Alliance
204 N. Chestnut Street
Kellogg, ID 83837
(208) 783-3535
fax: (208) 783-4848
email: info@reikialliance.com
website: www.reikialliance.com

## Relaxation/Meditation:
*Relaxation:*
American Psychiatric Association
1000 Wilson Blvd., Suite 1825
Arlington, VA 22209-3901
(888)35-PSYCH/(888) 357-7924
   or (703) 907-7300
website: www.psych.org

American Psychological
   Association
750 First Street, NE
Washington, DC 20002-4242
(800) 374-2721 or (202) 336-5510
website: www.apa.org

National Association of Social
   Workers
750 First Street, NE, Suite 700
Washington, DC 20002-4241
(800) 638-8799 or (202) 408-8600
website: www.naswdc.org

*Meditation:*
American Organization for
   Bodywork Therapies of Asia
   (AOBTA)
1010 Haddonfield-Berlin Road,
   Suite 408
Voorhees, NJ 08043-3514
(856) 782-1616

fax: (856) 782-1653
email: aobta@prodigy.net
website: www.aobta.org
(for tai chi and qigong)

International Association of Yoga
  Therapists (IAYT)
2400A County Center Drive
Santa Rosa, CA 95403
(707) 566-9000
email: mail@iayt.org
website: www.iayt.org
(IAYT is a special division of Yoga
  Research and Education Center)

Transcendental Meditation
(888) 532-7686
(This number will ring in the state
  from which you are calling. The
  operator will provide you with
  information on transcendental
  meditation instructors near you.)

**Rolfing:**
Rolf Institute
205 Canyon Boulevard
Boulder, CO 80302
(800) 530-8875 or (303) 449-5903
fax: (303) 449-5978
website: www.rolf.org

National Certification Board for
  Therapeutic Massage and
  Bodywork
8201 Greensboro Drive, Suite 300
McLean, VA 22102
(800) 296-0664 or (703) 610-9015
fax: (703) 610-9005
email: info@ncbtmb.com
website: www.ncbtmb.com

**Shiatsu:**
American Organization for
  Bodywork Therapies of Asia
  (AOBTA)
1010 Haddonfield-Berlin Road,
  Suite 408
Voorhees, NJ 08043-3514
(856) 782-1616
fax: (856) 782-1653
email: aobta@prodigy.net
website: www.aobta.org

National Certification Commission for Acupuncture and
  Oriental Medicine (NCCAOM)
11 Canal Center Plaza, Suite 300
Alexandria, VA 22314
(703) 548-9004
fax: (703) 548-9079
email: info@nccaom.org
website: www.nccaom.org

National Certification Board for
  Therapeutic Massage and
  Bodywork
8201 Greensboro Drive, Suite 300
McLean, VA 22102
(800) 296-0664 or (703) 610-9015
fax: (703) 610-9005
email: info@ncbtmb.com
website: www.ncbtmb.com

**Sports Massage:**
American Massage Therapy
  Association
820 Davis Street, Suite 100
Evanston, IL 60201
(847) 864-0123
fax: (847) 864-1178
website: www.amtamassage.org

National Certification Board for
  Therapeutic Massage and
  Bodywork
8201 Greensboro Drive, Suite 300
McLean, VA 22102
(800) 296-0664 or (703) 610-9015
fax: (703) 610-9005
email: info@ncbtmb.com
website: www.ncbtmb.com

**Swedish Massage:**
American Massage Therapy
  Association
820 Davis Street, Suite 100
Evanston, IL 60201
(847) 864-0123
fax: (847) 864-1178
website: www.amtamassage.org

National Certification Board for
  Therapeutic Massage and
  Bodywork
8201 Greensboro Drive, Suite 300
McLean, VA 22102
(800) 296-0664 or (703) 610-9015
fax: (703) 610-9005
email: info@ncbtmb.com
website: www.ncbtmb.com

**Tai Chi:**
American Organization for
  Bodywork Therapies of Asia
  (AOBTA)
1010 Haddonfield-Berlin Road,
  Suite 408
Voorhees, NJ 08043-3514
(856) 782-1616
fax: (856) 782-1653
email: aobta@prodigy.net
website: www.aobta.org

**Therapeutic Touch:**
Nurse Healers-Professional
  Associates International
3760 South Highland Drive,
  Suite 429
Salt Lake City, Utah 84106
(801) 273-3399
fax: (509) 693-3537
email: NH-PAI@Therapeutic-
  Touch.org
website: www.therapeutic-
  touch.org

**Traditional Chinese
Medicine:**
National Certification
  Commission for Acupuncture
  and Oriental Medicine
  (NCCAOM)
11 Canal Center Plaza,
  Suite 300
Alexandria, VA 22314
(703) 548-9004
fax: (703) 548-9079
email: info@nccaom.org
website: www.nccaom.org

Acupuncture and Oriental
  Medicine Alliance (AOMA)
6405 43rd Avenue Ct. NW,
  Suite B
Gig Harbor, WA 98335
(253) 851-6896
fax: (253) 851-6883
website: www.aomalliance.org

American Association of Oriental
  Medicine (AAOM)
5530 Wisconsin Avenue,
  Suite 1210

Chevy Chase, MD 20815
(888) 500-7999 or (301) 941-1064
fax: (301) 986-9313
email: info@aaom.org
website: www.aaom.org

**The Trager Approach:**
Trager Institute
21 Locust Avenue
Mill Valley, CA 94941
(415) 388-2688
fax: (415) 388-2710
email: admin@trager.com
website: www.trager.com

Trager International
24800 Chagrin Blvd., Suite 205
Beachwood, Ohio 44122
(216) 896-9383
email: trager@trager.com
website: www.trager.com

National Certification Board for
  Therapeutic Massage and
  Bodywork
8201 Greensboro Drive, Suite 300
McLean, VA 22102
(800) 296-0664 or (703) 610-9015
fax: (703) 610-9005
email: info@ncbtmb.com
website: www.ncbtmb.com

**Trigger Point Therapy:**
Bonnie Prudden Myotherapy
4330 East Havasu Road
Tucson, AZ 85718
(800) 221-4634 or (520) 529-3979
fax: (520) 529-6679
www.bonnieprudden.com

International Myotherapy
  Association
email: info@myotherapy.org
website: www.myotherapy.org

# Bibliography

Aihara, Cornelia, and Herman Aihara. *Natural Healing From Head to Toe: Traditional Macrobiotic Remedies.* Garden City Park, NY: Avery Publishing Group, 1994.

Alon, Ruthy. *Mindful Spontaneity: Lessons in the Feldenkrais Method.* Berkeley, CA: North Atlantic Books, 1994.

Altman, Nathaniel. *Everybody's Guide to Chiropractic Health Care.* Los Angeles: Jeremy P. Tarcher, Inc., 1990.

Antol, Marie Nadine. *Healing Teas: How to Prepare and Use Teas to Maximize Your Health.* Garden City Park, NY: Avery Publishing Group, 1996.

Anson, Brian. *Rolfing: Stories of Personal Empowerment.* Kansas City: Heartland Personal Growth Press, 1992.

Astor, Stephen. *Hidden Food Allergies: Finding the Foods That Cause You Problems and Removing Them From Your Diet.* Garden City Park, NY: Avery Publishing Group, 1997.

Aubin, Michel, and Philippe Picard. *Homeopathy & Your Health: A Different Way of Treating Common Everyday Ailments.* Garden City Park, NY: Avery Publishing Group, 1996.

Bach, Edward, M.D., and F.J. Wheeler. *The Bach Flower Remedies.* New Canaan, CT: Keats Publishing, Inc., 1979.

Baginski, Bodo J., and Shalila Sharaman. *Reiki: Universal Life Energy.* Mendocino, CA: Life Rhythm Publications, 1988.

Baker, Jan. *Yoga for Real People.* York Beach, ME: Red Wheel/Weiser, LLC, 2002

Balch, James F., M.D., and Phyllis A. Balch, C.N.C. *Prescription for Nutritional Healing.* Garden City Park, NY: Avery Publishing Group, 1996.

Bandler, Richard, and John Grinder. *Neuro-Linguistic Programming and the Transformation of Meaning.* Moab, UT: Real People Press, 1982.

Barnett, Libby and Chambers, Maggie. *Reiki Energy Medicine.* Rochester, VT: Healing Arts Press, 1996.

Beaulieu, John, N.D., Ph.D., R.P.P. *Polarity Therapy Workbook.* New York: BioSonic Enterprises, Ltd., 1994.

Beck, Mark F. *Milady's Theory and Practice of Therapeutic Massage.* 2d ed. Albany, NY: Milady Publishing Company, 1994.

Benjamin Patricia J. and Lamp Scott P. *Understanding Sports Massage.* Champaign, IL: Human Kinetics, 1996.

Benson, Herbert, M.D. *The Relaxation Response.* New York: Outlet Books, 1993.

Benson, Herbert, M.D., and Eileen M. Stuart, R.N., M.S. *The Wellness Book.* New York: Fireside, 1993.

Benson, Herbert, M.D., and Marg Stark. *Timeless Healing: The Power and Biology of Belief.* New York: Scribner, 1996.

Benson, Herbert, M.D., and William Proctor. *Your Maximum Mind.* New York: Times Books, 1987.

Beresford-Cooke, Carola, and Peter Albright. *Acupressure (Naturally Better).* New York: Quarto (Macmillan Information), 1996.

Berger, Stuart M., M.D. *How to be Your Own Nutritionist.* New York: William Morrow & Co., 1987.

Birch, Beryl Bender. *Power Yoga: The Total Strength and Flexibility Workout.* New York: Fireside, 1995.

Blumenfeld, Larry, ed. *The Big Book of Relaxation: Simple Techniques to Control The Excess Stress in Your Life.* Roslyn, NY: The Relaxation Company, 1994.

Blumenthal, Mark, Sr. Editor. *Herbal Medicine.* Newton, MA: Integrative Medicine Communications: 2000.

Bond, Mary. *Balancing Your Body: A Self-Help Approach to Rolfing Movement.* Rochester, VT: Inner Traditions International, Ltd., 1996.

Borysenko, Joan. *Minding the Body/Mending the Mind.* New York: Bantam Books, 1989.

Bourne, Edmund J., Ph.D. *The Anxiety and Phobia Workbook.* Oakland, CA: New Harbinger Publications, Inc., 1995.

Brody, Jane. *Jane Brody's Nutrition Book.* New York: Bantam Books, 1987.

Bruckner-Gordon, Fredda, D.S.W., Barbara Gangi, C.S.W., and Geraldine Waliman, D.S.W. *Making Therapy Work: Your Guide to Choosing, Using, and Ending Therapy.* New York: Harper & Row, 1988.

Burton Goldberg Group. *Alternative Medicine: The Definitive Guide.* Puyallup, WA: Future Medicine Publishing, Inc., 1993.

Carrico, Mara. *Yoga Basics: The Essential Beginners Guide to Yoga for a Lifetime of Health and Fitness.* New York: Henry Holt, 1997

Carter, Mildred, and Tammy Weber. *Healing Yourself with Foot Reflexology: All Natural Relief from Dozens of Ailments.* Englewood Cliffs, NJ: Prentice Hall, 1997.

Carter, Mildred. *Body Reflexology: Healing at Your Fingertips.* West Nyack, NY Parker Publishing Co., 1983.

Castleman, Michael. *The New Healing Herbs.* Rodale, Inc., 2001.

Chin, Richard, M.D., O.M.D. *The Energy Within: The Science Behind Every Oriental Therapy from Acupuncture to Yoga.* New York: Marlowe & Co., 1995.

Chopra, Deepak, M.D. *Perfect Health: The Complete Mind/Body Guide.* New York: Harmony Books, 1991.

Clark, Nancy. *Sports Nutrition Guidebook.* Champaign: Leisure Press, 1990.

Cohen, Dan. *An Introduction to CranioSacral Therapy: Anatomy, Function and Treatment.* Berkeley, CA: North Atlantic Books, 1995.

Cohen, Kenneth S. *The Way of Qigong.* New York: Ballantine Books, 1997.

Crayhon, Robert, M.S. *Nutrition Made Simple.* New York, NY: M. Evans & Co., Inc., 1996.

Danskin, David, Ph.D., and M. Crow, Ph.D. *Biofeedback: An Introduction and Guide.* Palo Alto, CA: Mayfield Publishing Co., 1981.

Davis, Martha, Ph.D., Elizabeth Robbins Eshelman, M.S.W., and Matthew McKay, Ph.D. *The Relaxation and Stress Reduction Workbook.* 4th ed. New York: New Harbinger Publications, Inc., 1995.

Ditts, Robert, Tim Hallbom, and Suzi Smith. *Beliefs: Pathways to Health and Well-Being.* Portland, OR: Metamorphosis Press, 1990.

Dossey, Larry, M.D. *Prayer is Good Medicine: How to Reap the Healing Benefit of Prayer.* New York: HarperCollins Publishers, 1996.

Dull, Harold. *WATSU: Freeing the Body in Water.* Middletown, CA: Harbin Springs Publ., 1993.

Eckert, Achim. *Chinese Medicine for Beginners: Use the Power of the Five Elements to Heal Body and Soul.* Rocklin, CA: Prima Publishing, 1996.

Eisenberg, David, M.D. *Encounters with Qi: Exploring Chinese Medicine 3rd edition.* New York: W.W. Norton, 1995.

Elinwood, Ellae. *The Everything T'ai Chi and Qigong Book.* Avon, MA: Adams Media Corp., 2002.

Feldenkrais, Moshe. *Awareness Through Movement: Health Exercises for Personal Growth.* San Francisco: Harper San Francisco, 1990.

Firebrace, Peter, and Sandra Hill. *Acupuncture: How It Works, How It Cures.* New Canaan, CT: Keats Publishing, 1994.

Fisher, Stanley, Ph.D. *Discovering the Power of Self-Hypnosis: The Simple Natural Mind-Body Approach to Change and Healing.* New York: Newmarket Press, 2000.

Gandee, William S., D.C., and Peggy Russell. *Triumph Over Illness: What You Should Know About the Power of Chiropractic Care.* Garden City Park, NY: Avery Publishing Group, 1997.

Gascoigne, Stephen, Dr. *The Chinese Way to Health: A Self-Help Guide to Traditional Chinese Medicine.* Boston, MA: Tuttle Publishing, 1997.

Gelb, Michael. *Body Learning: An Introduction to the Alexander Technique.* New York: H. Holt and Co., 1996.

Goldsmith, Joel S. *The Art of Meditation.* 2d ed. New York: HarperCollins Publishers, 1990.

Goodman, Saul. *The Book of Shiatsu: The Healing Art of Finger Pressure.* Garden City Park, NY: Avery Publishing Group, Inc., 1990.

Gordon, James S., M.D. *Stress Management.* New York: Chelsea House Publishers, 1990.

Hallowell, Michael. *Herbal Healing: A Practical Introduction to Medicinal Herbs.* Garden City Park, NY: Avery Publishing Group, Inc., 1994.

Harrison, Sheila. *Help Your Child With Homeopathy: Using Natural Homeopathic Remedies to Relieve Common Childhood Ailments.* Garden City Park, NY: Avery Publishing Group, 1996.

Hatcher, Chris, and Philip Himelstein, eds. *The Handbook of Gestalt Therapy.* Northvale, NJ: Jason Aronson, Inc., 1995.

Heussenstamm, Frances K., Ph.D. *Blame It On Freud: A Guide to the Language of Psychology.* Georgetown, MA: North Star Publications, 1993.

Houston, F.M. *Healing Benefits of Acupressure: Acupuncture without Needles.* 2d ed. New Canaan, CT: Keats Publishing, 1993.

Huang, Master Alfred. *Complete Tai Chi: The Definitive Guide to Physical and Emotional Self-Improvement.* Rutland, VT: Charles E. Tuttle Company, 1993.

Huey, Lynda, and Robert Forster, PT. *The Complete Waterpower Workout Book.* New York: Random House, 1993.

Hunervogt, Tanmaya. *The Power of Reiki.* New York, NY: Henry Holt and Co., Inc. 1998.

Ingham, Eunice D. *The Original Works of Eunice D. Ingham: Stories The Feet Can Tell and Stories The Feet Have Told.* St. Petersburg, FL: Ingham Publishing, Inc., 1984.

Jahnke, Roger. *The Most Profound Medicine.* Santa Barbara, CA: Health Action Books, 1990.

Jarmey, Chris and Mojay, Gabriel. *Shiatsu: The Complete Guide.* Hammersmith, London: Thorsons, 1991.

Jensen, Bernard, Dr. *Foods That Heal: A Guide to Understanding and Using the Healing Powers of Natural Foods.* Garden City Park, NY: Avery Publishing Group, 1993.

Johnson, Joan. *The Healing Art of Sports Massage.* Emmaus, PA: Rodale Press, Inc., 1995.

Kabat-Zinn, Jon, Ph.D. *Full Catastrophe Living: Using the Wisdom of Your Body and Mind to Face Stress, Pain and Illness.* New York: Bantam Doubleday Dell Publishing Group, Inc., 1990.

Kaptchuk, Ted, J. *The Web That Has No Weaver: Understanding Chinese Medicine.* New York: Congdon Weed, 1983.

Kaslof, Leslie J. *The Bach Remedies: A Self Help Guide.* New Canaan, CT: Keats Publishing, 1988.

Kean, Frances and Voorhees, Susan. *A Simple Guide to Yoga.* White Plains, NY: Peter Pauper Press, 2002.

Kenyon, Julian, M.D. *Acupressure Techniques: A Self-Help Guide.* Rochester, VT: Healing Arts Press, 1998.

Kogler, Aladar, Ph.D. *Yoga for Every Athlete.* St. Paul, MN: Llewellyn Publications, 1995.

Koury, Joanne M., M.Ed. *Aquatic Therapy Programming*. Champaign, IL: Human Kinetics, 1996.

Krasner, A.M., Ph.D. *The Wizard Within: The Krasner Method of Clinical Hypnotherapy*. Santa Ana, CA: American Board of Hypnotherapy Press, 1990.

Krieger, Dolores, Ph.D., R.N. *Accepting Your Power to Heal: Personal Practice of Therapeutic Touch*. Santa Fe, NM: Bear & Co., Inc., 1993.

Krieger, Dolores, Ph.D., R.N. *Therapeutic Touch Inner Workbook: Ventures in Transpersonal Healing*. Santa Fe, NM: Bear & Co., Inc., 1997.

Kushi, Michio. *The Macrobiotic Way*. Garden City Park, NY: Avery Publishing Group, 1993.

Lad, Vasant, B.A.M.S. *The Complete Book of Ayurvedic Home Remedies*. New York: Three Rivers Press, 1998.

Lawless, Julia. *The Encyclopedia of Essential Oils*. Rockport, MA: Element Books, Inc., 1993.

Leibowitz, Judith, and Bill Connington. *The Alexander Technique*. New York: HarperCollins Publishers, 1991.

Lockie, Andrew, Dr. *Natural Health Encyclopedia of Homeopathy*. New York: Dorling Kindersley, 2000.

Lowen, Alexander, M.D. *Bioenergetics*. New York: Penguin USA, 1994.

Lowen, Alexander, M.D. *Joy: The Surrender to the Body and to Life*. New York: Penguin USA, 1995.

MacDonald, Glynn. *Illustrated Elements of Alexander Technique*. Hammersmith, London: Element, 2002.

Macrae, Janet. *Therapeutic Touch: A Practical Guide*. New York: Alfred A. Knopf, 1988.

Mark, Bow-Sim. *Combined Tai Chi Chuan*. Boston: Chinese Wushu Research Institute, 1979.

Maxwell-Hudson, Clare. *Aromatherapy Massage*. New York: DK Publishing, Inc., 1997.

McCarty, Meredith. *American Macrobiotic Cuisine*. Garden City Park, NY: Avery Publishing Group, 1996.

McCarty, Patrick. *The Beginner's Guide to Shiatsu: Using Japanese Finger*

*Pressure for the Relief of Headaches, Back Pain, and Hypertension.* Garden City Park, NY: Avery Publishing Group, Inc., 1995.

McDermott, Ian, and Joseph O'Connor. *Neuro-Linguistic Programming and Health.* San Francisco: Thorsons, 1996.

McGee, Charles T., M.D., and Master Effie Poy Yew Chow. *Qigong: Miracle Healing from China.* Coeur d'Alene, ID: MediPress, 1994.

McGill, Leonard. *The Chiropractor's Health Book: Simple, Natural Exercises for Relieving Headaches, Tension and Back Pain.* New York: Crown Publishing, Inc., 1997.

Meagher, Jack, and Pat Boughton. *Sports Massage: A Complete Program for Increasing Performance and Endurance in 15 Popular Sports.* Barrytown, NY: Station Hill Press, 1990.

Miller, Lyle H., Ph.D., Anna Smith, Ph.D., and Larry Rothstein, Ed.D. *The Stress Solution.* New York: Simon and Schuster, Inc., 1993.

Morrison, Judith H. *The Book of Ayurveda: A Holistic Approach to Health and Longevity.* New York: Fireside, 1995.

Muller, Brigitte, and Horst H. Gunther. *A Complete Book of Reiki Healing.* Mendocino, CA: Life Rhythm Publications, 1995.

Mumford, Susan. *The Complete Guide to Massage: A Step by Step Approach to Total Body Relaxation.* New York: Plume (Penguin Group), 1996.

Murray, Michael, N.D., and Joseph Pizzorno, N.D. *Encyclopedia of Natural Medicine.* Rocklin, CA: Prima Publishing, 1991.

Naparstek, Belleruth. *Staying Well with Guided Imagery: How to Harness the Power of Your Imagination for Health and Healing.* New York: Warner Books, 1994.

Nevis, Edwin C., ed. *Gestalt Therapy: Perspectives and Applications.* New York: Gardner Press, Inc., 1992.

O'Connor, John, and Dan Bensky. *Acupuncture: A Comprehensive Text.* Chicago: Eastland Press, 1981.

Ody, Penelope. *The Holistic Herbal Directory.* Edison, NJ: Chartwell Books, Inc., 2001.

Paris, Bob. *Natural Fitness: Your Complete Guide to a Healthy, Balanced System.* New York: Warner Books, 1996.

Parsa-Stay, Flora, D.D.S. *The Complete Book of Dental Remedies: A Guide to*

*Safe and Effective Relief from the Most Common Dental Problems Using Homeopathy, Natural Supplements, Herbs, and Conventional Dental Care.* Garden City Park, NY: Avery Publishing Group, 1996.

Patterson Wildemann, Ann. *Sessions: A Self-Help Guide Through Psychotherapy.* New York: The Crossroad Publishing Company, 1996.

Peper, Erik, and Catherine Holt. *Creating Wholeness: A Self-Healing Workbook Using Dynamic Relaxation, Images and Thoughts.* New York: Plenum Publishing Group, 1993.

Pierrakos, John C., M.D. *Core Energetics: Developing the Capacity to Love and Heal.* Mendocino, CA: Life Rhythm Pub., 1987.

Prudden, Bonnie. *Myotherapy: Bonnie Prudden's Complete Guide to Pain Free Living.* 2d ed. New York: The Dial Press, 1984.

Prudden, Bonnie. *Pain Erasure: The Bonnie Prudden Way.* New York: Ballantine Books, 1985.

Reader's Digest Association. *Magic and Medicine of Plants.* Pleasantville, NY: Reader's Digest Association, Inc., 1986.

Rolf, Ida P. *Rolfing and Physical Reality.* Rochester, VT: Healing Arts Press, 1990.

Rolf, Ida P. *Rolfing: Re-establishing the Natural Alignment and Structural Integration of the Human Body for Health and Vitality.* Rochester, VT: Healing Arts Press, 1989.

Rossman, Martin L., M.D. *Guided Imagery for Self-Healing.* Tiburon, CA: H.J. Kramer, 2000.

Ruoti, Richard G., David M. Morris, Andrew J. Cole. *Aquatic Rehabilitation.* New York: Lippincott Raven Publishers, 1996.

Samskrti and Veda. *Hatha Yoga: Manual 1.* 2d ed. Honesdale, PA: The Himalayan International Institute of Yoga Science and Philosophy of the U.S.A., 1986.

Seidman, Maruti. *A Guide To Polarity Therapy: The Gentle Art of Hands-On Healing.* Boulder: Elan Press, 1991.

Shafarman, Steve. *Awareness Heals: The Feldenkrais Method for Dynamic Health.* Reading, MA: Addison-Wesley, 1997.

Sharon, Michael, Dr. *Complete Nutrition.* Garden City Park, NY: Avery Publishing Group, 1989.

Singh, Rajinder. *Inner and Outer Peace Through Meditation.* Rockport, MA: Element Books, Inc., 1996.

So Tin Yau, James, Dr. *The Book of Acupuncture Points.* Brookline, MA: Paradigm Publications, 1985.

Stone, Randolph. *Polarity Therapy: The Complete Collected Works, Volume I and II.* Sebastopol, CA: CRCS Publications, 1986.

Tappen, Frances M., Ed.D, M.A. *Healing Massage Techniques.* 3rd ed. Norwalk: Appleton & Lange, 1998.

Tousley, Dirk, and David M. Lees. *The Chiropractic Handbook for Patients.* Independence, MO: White Dove Publishing Co., 1985.

Trager, Milton, MD., and Cathy Hammond. *Movement as a Way to Agelessness: A Guide to Trager Mentastics.* Barrytown, NY: Station Hill Press, 1995.

Ullman, Dana. *Homeopathy A-Z.* Carlsbad, CA: Hay House, Inc., 1999.

Ullman, Dana. *The Consumer's Guide to Homeopathy: The Definitive Resource for Understanding Homeopathic Medicine and Making It Work For You.* New York: Jeremy P. Tarcher, Inc., 1996.

Upledger, John E., D.O., F.A.A.O. *Your Inner Physician and You: Cranio-Sacral Therapy, Somato-Emotional Release.* Berkeley, CA: North Atlantic Books, 1997.

Vishnudevananda, Swami. *The Complete Illustrated Book of Yoga.* New York: Harmony Books, 1980.

Walberg, L.R. *Hypnosis: Is it for You?* New York: Dembner Books, 1982.

Walsh, William, M.D., F.A.C.A. *The Food Allergy Book.* Garden City Park, NY: Avery Publishing Group, 1995.

Weil, Andrew, M.D. *Natural Health Natural Medicine.* New York: Houghton Mifflin, 1998.

Weiner, Michael, Dr. *The Complete Book of Homeopathy: The Holistic and Natural Way to Good Health.* Garden City Park, NY: Avery Publishing Group, 1996.

Whichello Brown, Denise. *Reflexology Basics.* New York: Sterling Publishing Co., Inc., 2001.

Wildwood, Christine. *Flower Remedies: Natural Healing with Flower Essences.* Rockport, MA: Element, 1995.

Wildwood, Chrissie. *The Encyclopedia of Aromatherapy.* Rochester, VT: Healing Arts Press, 1996.

Wilk, Chester A., D.C. *Medicine, Monopolies and Malice: How the Medical Establishment Tried to Destroy Chiropractic in the U.S.* Garden City Park, NY: Avery Publishing Group, 1996.

Williams, Tom. *Chinese Medicine.* Rockport, MA: Element Books, 1997.

Williamson, Vivien. *Bach Remedies and Other Flower Essences.* New York, NY: Lorenz Books, Anness Publishing, Inc.: 2000.

Wilson, Roberta. *Aromatherapy for Vibrant Health and Beauty: A Practical A to Z Reference to Aromatherapy Treatments for Health, Skin, and Hair Problems Using Essential Oils.* Garden City Park, NY: Avery Publishing Group, 1995.

Wise, Anna. *The High-Performance Mind: Mastering Brainwaves for Insight, Healing and Creativity.* Putnam, NY: Jeremy P. Tarcher, Inc., 1995.

Yamamoto, Shizuko, and Patrick McCarty. *The Shiatsu Handbook: A Guide to the Traditional Art of Shiatsu Acupressure.* Garden City Park, NY: Avery Publishing Group, 1996.

# Index

Muscle pain, 25, 29, 75, 84, 128, 136, 140, 161. *See also* Musculoskeletal disorders.
Muscle tone, 141, 145
Muscular cramps, 22, 43, 59, 99.
Muscular dystrophy, 156. *See also* Musculoskeletal disorders.
Musculoskeletal disorders, 34, 39, 52, 67, 93, 104, 120, 128, 136, 140, 161
Myotherapy, 88. *See also* Trigger Point Therapy.

Naturopathy, 88–92. *See also* Acupuncture; Exercise; Herbal Medicine; Homeopathy; Hydrotherapy; Nutritional Counseling; Osteopathy; Psychotherapy; Traditional Chinese Medicine.
Nausea, 29, 59, 93, 100
Neck pain, 12, 17, 22, 43, 48, 99, 128, 132, 140, 156
Needle therapy. *See* Acupuncture.
Nerve, pinched, 22, 128
Nervous system disorders, 34, 67, 120, 141, 145, 148
Nervous tension. *See* Emotional health disorders.
Neuralgia, 12, 17, 43, 60, 140
Neuritis. *See* Nervous system disorders.
Neurolinguistic programming (NLP), 107–108
Neurological injuries, 25
Neuromuscular disorders, 85, 140
NLP. *See* Neurolinguistic programming.
Norcross, John, 107
Nose problems, 22, 29, 34, 67, 93
Numbness, 161

Nutritional Counseling, 92–98. *See also* Ayurveda; Traditional Chinese Medicine.

Obesity, 25, 79, 93
Oriental nutrition, 95
Orthopedic problems, 25. *See also* Musculoskeletal disorders.
Osteoarthritis, 157. *See also* Musculoskeletal disorders.
Osteopathy, 47, 90
Overuse syndromes, 161

Pain, chronic, 25, 29, 39, 60, 75, 104, 113, 116, 128, 136, 149, 161
Palmer, Bartlett Joshua, 42
Palmer, Daniel David, 42
Palmer Infirmary and Chiropractic Institute, 42
Panic, 104, 113, 145. *See also* Anxiety; Emotional health disorders.
Parkinson's disease, 93
Pattern of disharmony, 152
Pelvic inflammatory disease (PID), 17
Pelvic pain, 12, 132
Perls, Frederick, 106
Personal training, 51. *See also* Nutritional Counseling.
Petrissage, 141
Phobias. *See* Emotional health disorders; Fears.
Phobias, dental, 71, 79. *See also* Hypnotherapy.
PID. *See* Pelvic inflammatory disease.
Pierreko, John, 106
Pitta, 35
PMS. *See* Premenstrual syndrome.
Polar energetics, 100–101